12 YEARS AFTER 7 MONTHS TO LIVE

12 YEARS AFTER 7 MONTHS TO LIVE

The Faith to Fight a Terminal Brain Tumor

CHARLIE AND SHERRI MARENGO

Broom Closet Studios

JAMES 5:13-16

Is anyone among you suffering? Let him pray. Is anyone cheerful? Let him sing praise. Is anyone among you sick? Let him call for the elders of the church, and let them pray over him, anointing him with oil in the name of the Lord. And the prayer of faith will save the one who is sick, and the Lord will raise him up. And if he has committed sins, he will be forgiven. Therefore, confess your sins to one another and pray for one another, that you may be healed. The prayer of a righteous person has great power as it is working.

~For Chivonne~ she was stronger than she thought~

"Have you ever been to the Grand Canyon?" he asked. This is the kind of 'bucket list' question that comes with a terminal brain tumor diagnosis. We are writing all this down to shed some light on the effects of a brain tumor diagnosis not just for the patient, but for the caregiver, the family, the friends. We also want to share some hope that if you are ever in this situation, something from this book will stand out to help you get through! Every case is different. Ours is unusual because the diagnosis of glioblastoma multiforme is almost always a sure and swift death sentence, and yet —here we are. If not for the big faith of our family, friends and church, as well as the excellent medical professionals on this case, the final outcome of this story might have been totally different. Our prayer is that through this personal journey you will see some hope you might not have known was there for you.

In His Service, Charlie and Sherri Marengo

REVIEWS

EARLY REVIEWS FOR "12 YEARS AFTER 7 MONTHS TO LIVE"

I do not put words on paper nearly as well as you. But first just let me say thank you for letting me preview your book.... for your willingness to put it all in print...... for the kind words written about my daddy...... for the encouragement y'all are giving to all who will read your story. You are both such an inspiration on trusting God! Praise the Lord for His wondrous love and grace and for the miracles He continues to manifest in our lives. I will continue to pray for y'all but more diligently now that I have a little more insight into your circumstances. We are told to run the race with endurance and your book gives evidence of your obedience. May God richly bless you for your good service to Him and continue to provide for your every need. **KAY BULLEN-GARRARD**

I must tell you that you both did an incredible job of putting your hearts on the table. Honesty, fears, faithfulness, tears and giving God the Glory. You've got a way with words, but Charlie is a wordsmith (as well as a Breadman). And I loved the connection with your journals. Great advice. I was brought to tears and feel really humbled to need to stop and look around me again and see the situations people are in that we are sometimes so unaware of - and just help someone breathe. Your "just tossed in" statements of advice are actually as engrossing and helpful as your list of sources at the end. And yours and Charlie's scriptural references will reach the audience that needs them when they are presented with them at the time their hearts are ready for them. Thanks for being Faithful. **ROBBIE LITTLE**

It's heartbreaking, emotional, inspiring, well worded, a page turner, amazing – I'm truly impressed! I think it's awesome the raw feelings, the ups and downs, the compassion, the faith is truly inspiring, sorry can't help it, it truly is awesome. Thank you for sharing this with me. This book was an inspirational, yet heartbreaking, emotional roller coaster. The faith this family has and the passages they share are so heartwarming. I couldn't put this book down, I had to read every word! When you open this book to read it, be prepared to get lost in its pages. **RITA PIEROTTI**

What a compelling and inspiring story! You and Charlie's strength during tough times is a testimony to us all. This book is a must-read for anyone needing a bit of encouragement to help them make it through the tough times. **Johnny Dupree, PhD, former Mayor of Hattiesburg MS**

I have finished your book and reread several parts of it. As God would have it the timing was perfect for my own life. It is riveting and inspiring. Overall it was an excellent, inspiring read. The journal excerpts were noteworthy. Much like a good sermon, it will touch many people in their hours of need when it is more widely available. I applaud you two for the effort and look forward to purchasing my personal published copy. Thank you for sharing with me. May God bless you both. We pray for wisdom, courage and strength. **Dr. Stephen Beam, MD**

TABLE OF CONTENTS

Dedication

I don't think this book would have even come from our hearts to the page if the two of us hadn't been 'stuck' together during a pandemic. As hard as it was to re-live some of these times, it helped and healed us as we looked back. The Thank you list is long enough to have its own chapter, but let us begin with our church families from Calvary Baptist Church in Petal, Grace Temple Ministries of Hattiesburg and, of course, Petal Harvey Baptist Church. Thank you to our children for growing up into fantastic adults and being there for us. We still pray for you by name every day. Thanks to Robyn Jackson for the guidance and editing info, even though she didn't live to read the finished product; to Robbie Little and Lucy Shows for their editing skills; to Vicki Baylis for the encouragement and the occasional casserole; My BFF's Blondie and Debra Jean for listening to me jabber on and on; to the ladies in my Sunday school class, The Sister Sharpeners, for praying without ceasing; and to the very breath in my lungs, the heartbeat of my soul, my husband - who truly is a WALKING MIRACLE. I thank my Savior Jesus Christ every day and night for allowing me to keep him.

Sherri

FORWARD BY DR. DUSTIE DUNN

When everything else fails, God doesn't. That message is simple to hear, but not easy to learn. In *12 Years After 7 Months to Live*, Charlie and Sherri Marengo tell a story that so many people, too many people, are facing. Cancer is no respecter of persons and it admits people into a club they never even considered joining. Through the ups and downs, God is faithful.

I'm so proud of the transparency that this book offers. Often forgotten, from the outside looking in, is that toll that cancer takes on the family and friends of the patient. This book lets the reader inside the mind and journey of those who live with cancer and those who love them. This is an important book for several reasons, but maybe at the top of the list is that here we find God at work in the day-to-day pressures of sickness.

Where medicine fails to know precisely how long, how severe, or how to move forward... God is not so limited. Medicine may not know what tomorrow will bring, but God sees even until 12 Years After 7 Months to live.

Dr. Dustie Dunn, Petal-Harvey Baptist Church, Petal, MS

CHAPTER 1

In the beginning... Meet the family

IN THE BEGINNING....

Sherri's story: I was born in Hattiesburg, Mississippi and spent half of first grade here before my family moved to San Antonio, Texas. I had one younger brother, and then a baby brother came along. My stepdad was an Army brat so he was used to moving. My mother liked adventure, evidently, so we spent several years there with my dad's family before moving back to Hattiesburg. The few 'kid' years in San Antonio were fun, for sure. Youngest brother Chris was always into something and, because our parents worked so much, I tried to keep him from losing limbs and falling out of trees and jumping off houses with umbrellas. My Mother would nearly faint at the sight of blood, so that time when Chris was in about 2nd grade and tried to slice off his thumb with a pocket knife, it was up to me to get help on the phone. Thank goodness my favorite aunt was a lifelong operating room nurse, and she could handle anything! I think being responsible for my baby brother helped me become a good caretaker later in life.

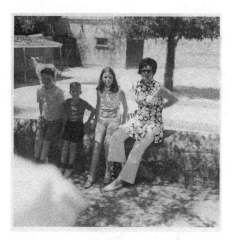

Brothers Nick and Chris with me and Mom at
the San Antonio Zoo 1969

He wasn't the only one accident prone, though, because I had my share of sprains and breaks. Just to highlight a few: fell off the pump house roof and cut my elbow on barbed wire fence at age seven; sprained my left ankle (the first time) falling off the bike; sprained my left ankle (the second time) skating on the street; cracked a rib getting dumped by a horse. And the best break of all? My13th birthday party at the skating rink. I was from the roller derby capital of the world in Texas so, yes, I raced on skates.

On that memorable day when I was flying low on eight wheels, someone hit me from behind, sending me into the concrete wall. When I opened my eyes, I was sitting with my back against the wall and seeing stars. The scary part was seeing everyone else looking at my wrists. Broken. Both wrists... broken. The ref rolled me to the office, where my mother promptly tried to faint, and I told them to call Aunt Myrna. She put my mangled arms on a pillow, covered me with ice bags and set up a surgery. That was not the most fun year of school ever with one cast to my elbow, one up to my shoulder. The old saying goes:

if you break everything as a kid, you are less likely to break stuff when you're an adult. Well, I'm glad I got that out of the way!

Back in Hattiesburg, I went to fourth grade at one school, fifth grade at another, and then we moved AGAIN to Texas. We stayed in one house for a record four years before coming back to Mississippi. By this time, I was in high school and ready to get out on my own.

I was used to being active and knew I was supposed to grow up and be a singer and radio DJ. Music is my life. When I wasn't with a band, I was singing with a traveling country music show based in Tupelo, Mississippi. I took a week's vacation in Memphis with some girls from the band, we found the Navy training base in Millington, TN and there were so many sailors to choose from that I did!

"Rick" and I married at the Justice of the Peace office in my hometown. Then we got stationed at NAS Pensacola for three years. In January 1978, his ship went to 'dry dock' in Pennsylvania. I flew to L.A. to stay with his family for three months. It was a nightmare that I won't detail, but the one great thing that happened was meeting a girl at work who took me to her church.

I got saved at Calvary Chapel in Downey, California, in February that year. It was the only way I stayed sane until I could get back to Florida. I promptly got pregnant and had a baby girl in December. Through a series of unfortunate events after that, I left with baby and dog and laundry and came home to my grandparents. That's where I was almost two years later when I met Charlie.

I was working a morning job at an employment office, afternoons on the local AM Country radio station and playing in a band at night. Not much time to sleep in between. I was doing an 'on location' radio gig the day Charlie walked into the Sunflower grocery store as a breadman for Colonial Bakery. I left a note on the bread truck, but it was two weeks later before we even knew each other's names.

He was also musically gifted, so he joined the band. And then we joined after only five months of knowing each other. We married in 1981 in Hattiesburg, Mississippi. Our wedding was in the living room of the rental house with just our family in attendance. A decade later, we had a full-blown church wedding to make up for the first one, with our children as our best man and maid of honor.

When we got married, we both had 2 ½ year old daughters from previous marriages, and then we had a son. Life was pretty smooth and certainly busy during the 80s. There was one exception to that: my near-death experience in March 1984. Writing this down now is almost as painful as it was that year.

As the first female program director at a local radio station, I answered to most of what the management asked of me. When it came time to let someone go that hadn't lived up to the job, they asked me to break the news. It didn't go over well. There was yelling, stomping, and threats before this person was asked to leave the property. After a couple of days, I just put it out of my mind, so I didn't make any connection to this scene with what would happen a week or so later.

Charlie was still on the bread truck and left the apartment at 4:30-ish every morning. It was Monday, March 19th. A hard blow to my head woke me out of a dead sleep. For that split second, I thought something had fallen off the wall. But two more blows came—hard and fast—as I turned my face into the pillow and screamed for Charlie. Of course, he was already gone to work, and in my total panic I jumped out of bed and ran down the hall toward the front door.

In a duplex, the bedrooms and bathrooms are usually separated by a wall from the kitchen/ living room. I came out of that dark hall to the front door, stepped out on the tiny porch and whistled. Like Ellie May Clampett, I whistled. Reflex? Maybe. But I also suddenly realized I was outside, so I jumped back in and slammed the door, locking the knob and the chain. I felt something warm on my shoulder and registered blood, a lot of blood. It was coming out of my right temple. Grabbing a kitchen towel, I held it over the wound and picked up the phone. Police? Ambulance? Charlie? I couldn't decide, so I dialed 0.

Operator: How may I help you?

Me: I need an ambulance, the police and my husband. I think someone tried to kill me.

O: Is the person still there? What's your address, ma'am? Is there anyone else there with you?

I gave her the address.

O: Where is your husband?

Me: He's at work at Colonial Bakery, in Hattiesburg.

O: The police and paramedics are on the way. Stand by.

I could hear clicking and another ring.

CB: Colonial.

Me: Tell Charlie he has to come home. Right now.

CB: Hang on. (in the distance- "Marengo!")

I honestly do not remember if he came to the phone. I felt a tug on my gown and looked down to see my daughter, age five, wide eyed and scared to death by what she saw.

"Momma, the baby's crying."

I slammed the phone down and ran back to the hallway to his room. When I flipped the light on, our two-year-old was standing up in the crib, crying at full volume. The window was OPEN. There was a short table with plastic figurines and baby toys on it below the sill. Everything had been tossed to the floor. Somehow, I held in the scream, picked up the baby and went back to the kitchen. I remember getting a bottle of milk out of the fridge. The knock on the door made my heart jump, so I opened it just a tiny bit, keeping the chain in place. Thank God, it was a Hattiesburg police officer.

HPD: Ma'am, it's okay. We're here to help.

Me: Okay, wait right here. I'm going to open the door, but don't come in. Just wait.

I put the kids on the couch and turned on the cartoons. This is evidently what people do when they're in shock. Our poor kids. They didn't make a sound. I motioned to the officer to come on in as I sat down at the dining room table, still clutching the bloody towel to my head. I could hear sirens getting closer, but before the ambulance could pull up, screeching tires told me Charlie had pulled in.

He ran in the house, took one look at the scene and almost lost it. I couldn't talk. I let the shock take over as he called my mom and checked on the children. The EMT's came in and it was a crowded house, for sure. Before I could be taken to the hospital, I insisted on changing clothes. After all, I couldn't possibly go to the emergency room in my nightgown!

Charlie walked me down the hall, and that's when we both saw the streaks of blood on the white wall—all the way from the bedroom to the front foyer. When he turned on the bedroom light for me to get some clothes, I saw myself in the mirror. Dear God. It was the stuff of nightmares. I was wearing a floor length white tee shirt that was now drenched in blood. My hair was a mess, and the blood was still coming out of the hole in my head. That's when I cried.

He helped peel off the gown and tossed it in the tub, wiped my face with a washcloth, found me a sweatshirt and some pants and helped me back down the hall where I allowed the paramedic to load me on the gurney.

The ride to Forrest General Hospital was filled with my anger. The attack was personal. The person who did this could have killed my kids! I was so mad that I railed on through the sobs. The hole in my head was just above my temple, which is why the blood kept spurting with every heartbeat. Sometimes God puts the right person in your path at the weirdest times, and for that, I was grateful to have an EMT named Danny Wiggins talking to me the entire ride. He was calm and had a steady hand, all the while telling me to take a breath and try to calm down so the wound would slow bleeding. We've remained friends ever since.

It was a square shaped wound and couldn't be sewn, so the doc packed it and covered it. While I was getting treated, Charlie made it to the hospital. He was as angry as I was, but, as men tend to do, he took it out on a concrete post, breaking his hand in the process.

That's when law enforcement decided he was the one that had tried to kill me. They never found any fingerprints or footprints as it was raining that morning. The whole incident became ridiculous. The media wouldn't report it because the police deemed it 'domestic'. That's another story for another day.

We left the hospital and went to my grandparent's house, where we stayed until we could find a rental house in the area. We slept with the kids between us in my Mama's king-sized bed. I was on heavy drugs for panic attacks and couldn't be left alone for even a minute. My mother and Charlie went back to the duplex to clean and pack. I never set foot back there. She moved in with us so I could have a babysitter until I was able to function again.

I quit that radio job. After six months of being scared to go from room to room in my own house, I had to get out. I got a job as a news chick with a funny morning show at a local rock radio station. Life got better, and I became an advocate for crime victims. We didn't talk about 'the incident' any more for years.

Working in radio was all I had done for years, but an opportunity came to me to move up to local TV news. In September 1985, Hurricane Elena traveled through the warm Gulf of Mexico waters to hit Biloxi as a Category 3 storm. The same night it hit the Mississippi coast, my baby brother Chris was in a near fatal auto accident. Our whole family was at the hospital with him all night, praying he would live after being thrown through the glass T-top of his car and up against a house. His skull was fractured horribly, but they wrapped it the best they could and waited for the neurosurgeon to make a decision. We stayed as long as we could, finally going home for sleep before returning the next morning.

That's when I got an unexpected call.

WDAM: "Are you still interested in this news position?"

Me: "Yes, of course. When do you need me?"

WDAM: "Be ready to roll in an hour, I have a cameraman coming to get you and he will brief you on the way to the coast. We need someone to cover the hurricane."

Um—okay!

I was ready in an hour. And clueless! I was so grateful to the veteran cameraman who gave me advice and tips all the way to the coast and set everything up for me to look real smart doing an interview with the Emergency Operations Director.

This was the way my career started as an anchor, producer, investigative reporter and bureau chief for a small market television station and later, news director for a cable news company. Charlie was 100% supportive of my job and crazy hours. Being naturally inquisitive (read that: nosey) sure came in handy later in life when I had to face the medical profession.

~~~~~

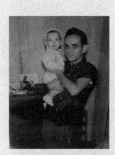

Al Sr. holding 'Jr' aka
Charlie

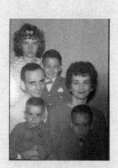

Faye, Charlie, Dad and
Mom, Martin and Chris

Charlie's story: I was raised in Gulfport, Mississippi, the oldest of three boys and two girls. My baby sister came along in 1965 on the heels of Hurricane Betsy. Mom and Dad could have named her Betsy but instead chose Dawn Michelle. I always liked the Dawn part of her name because it made me think of the beginning of a new day.

Not too many years later, I protected my baby sister from a deadly garden snake. As I was pushing her up the sidewalk to the house, a snake crossed our path, so I saved my sis from the evil green MONSTER and yelled for mom to kill the beast! To a nine-year-old, this venomous creature was ready to devour my sister and me. I did my best to be the oldest brother and protector of the youngest child.

Both of my sisters left impressions on me- but in completely opposite ways. Michelle was sweet and bright. My older sister was neither of those. She was the one who beat the daylights out of me when at age nine I packed my sack lunch and decided I was running away from home. I got about six blocks away before she caught me and beat me with a flip-flop all the way home, for what felt like twelve blocks. I have never forgotten that day. She warned me, with a few expletives, that if I ever tried something like that again I might not live to regret it!

We moved across the street from a church that would have a lasting effect on our entire family. By 1971, every one of us would become born again Christians. As for what the future would hold, only God knew, and has proven His faithfulness repeatedly. Dad was the last one in the family to come to Christ. Dad's passion and enthusiasm would dramatically change him forever, and he became so involved that he taught children's church. I remember one time he taught the story of David and Goliath. Dad's description of David was the equivalent of a "surfer-dude." It went something like this: "David was muscular, long blonde hair, powerful hands from slinging stones and killing lions." Somehow, I have the idea that he was describing David as pictured in a children's book.

Dad was the third of five boys and two girls of Italian descent. The family was hardworking, and their father died before most of the children reached their teens. Our grandmother remarried a Navy veteran who raised the children as his own. Perhaps this influenced my Dad. When he and mom met in 1955, not only did he take a future bride but a little blonde girl eight years old. He raised her as his own. Faye was a typical teenager in the 60s, a lover of rock-n-roll and fast cars. She suffered brain damage in a near-fatal car accident at age fifteen; it affected her personality as she grew older, but she never stopped being overly protective of her brothers. Widowed now, she lives a reclusive life in a small town in Alabama.

In 1956, Mom and Dad welcomed me as their first child and by 1959, had added two more boys to the mix. Martin and Chris were as different as night and day. Times were hard for a family of five back then. We lived in rentals that barely allowed enough space for three boys in one room. Bathroom time was limited, and our bedroom had just enough clearance between beds.

We spent one summer with our grandparents, who taught us respect, manners, and discipline. Papa was a navy veteran and did not tolerate our lack of manners, so every time "yes" wasn't followed by "sir" all three of us were disciplined. In fact, should one of us disobey or get out of line, all of us suffered his correction. Thinking back on it now, his military manner of discipline taught us structure and correction that is priceless.

Dad was offered a job at Colonial Baking Company in 1956. His stepfather helped build the Bakery after WWII, and after they completed the building, many of the workers were offered positions at the plant. Dad started in the production department. By the mid to late 70s, he became the foreman of the production department. With only an 8th grade education, Dad had a mathematical skill to be envied. There was not a formula or problem that he encountered in terms of time to produce bread or change needed for unfavorable conditions that he could not immediately scribble on paper and apply.

His dedication and commitment were at its best the night that Hurricane Camille came in 1969. He managed the entire department to produce the most loaves of bread in a 24-hour period until the storm knocked out the power and blew in a window. I can remember vividly Dad walking in the door that night, bringing calm in the middle of a loud and howling hurricane outside.

The next morning some friends came over on bicycles and we pedaled the two miles to the beach to see what, to my recollection, was complete destruction. As a 13-year-old kid, I was oblivious to any danger or potential hazard around us. We made our way through so much mud and debris that the only thing we could see was a GIGANTIC BOAT lying across the highway. And drink machines. Drink machines! Hallelujah, we've hit the jackpot—free sodas! When we got back home, we divided the spoils and made a pact to never tell a soul. But I guess it's a little too late for that now!

The friends and relationships made during my teen years would last a lifetime. Two classmates, one a next-door neighbor and the other a friend I met at church, would eventually become college roommates. Jimmy was the kind of guy who would be there whenever you needed him. If you were in a bind at 2:00 in the morning, he was that friend. Gary was unassuming, and always eager to listen and offer advice. We would spend nights together learning songs from Christian music groups. Gary and I played guitar and, remarkably, the three of us had pretty good voices, although our guitar skills would not improve for years. We were deeply involved at our church and high school.

Eventually, Gary and I would serve as traveling weekend guests at several churches throughout our junior college years. Those days were some of the best times of our lives. Gary met his wife on campus, and my first wife was her roommate. The four of us stayed on the road most weekends and rarely got to go home to visit family. After graduation, we went our separate ways. Jimmy went back to our hometown after one semester at college and married into the military. Gary returned to his hometown for a while and ended up in Arkansas for a brief time at his uncle's manufacturing plant. After completing his seminary degree, they made Arkansas home.

Gary and I married the same year and went on to serve in different locations in ministry. We had daughters born the same year. Our lives would not serve in the same capacity as we thought life would take us. Gary served as pastor for decades, and without a doubt he was blessed with the personality and obvious maturity early in life to be such. I felt like I was in a foreign land with no direction or purpose. I had no idea what I was doing. I felt doubt and feared failure, and my closest friend was hundreds of miles away. In less than two years, my service in that church was over, and Gary, always Mr. Dependable, helped us move from Winona back to Gulfport.

Prior to this move, they diagnosed my baby sister Michelle with bone cancer. She was a super active little girl, a cheerleader, a Brownie, and had dreams of being a gymnast. Michelle complained about her leg hurting her, but my parents thought it was just growing pains. The specifics of her diagnosis, treatment options, and other issues that cancer patients and parents have to make are vague to me, because of distance and obligations, but mostly just life. Michelle died just shy of her 14th birthday from the effects of osteosarcoma. Many times, survivors die from treatment effects rather than cancer's trauma on the body.

After Michelle's death, my parents were given some comfort through their time with my daughter. It may seem somewhat odd, but perhaps it is not anything more than God's provision in times of grief that when one child is lost, another is provided to calm the seas.

The death of my sister troubled me concerning my children, not myself or other siblings. It took me almost 20 years to come to terms with her death. My younger brother is the only one who experienced our mother's grief and sorrow from the initial diagnosis to Michelle's death. I cannot imagine losing a child, but watching cancer destroy a life you brought into this world has to be the worst loss of all! When my mother got the news of my diagnosis, she assured me she had a personal talk to God about it. Whether your child is 14 or 52, it really doesn't matter, because your children are supposed to outlive you. The thought of leaving my children, grandchildren, brothers, and Sherri behind is beyond comprehension. This is the reality of a disease. But the point is—you don't want to outlive your kids. It's the natural order of life. Moreover, it's the very impetus for the desire to LIVE!

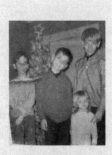

Martin, Chris, Charlie
and Michelle, the 60s

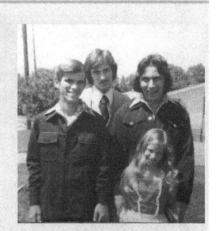

Martin, Charlie,
Chris and
Michelle, the 70s

My father helped me find a job as a salesperson for Colonial. I was now a "Breadman". The 70 mile drive everyday put added stress on life and relationships. My day began at 3am and ended at 11pm. The work was time-consuming and demanding but financially rewarding. I had only had two jobs up to this point. While in college, I worked at a national grocery store and as a teen for a stone mason contractor from our church. The things I learned from Ernie Bullen, known as Mr. B., would become a benchmark for my life and career as a salesman. When I was 15, at church on a Wednesday night, he walked up behind me, put his hands on my skinny shoulders and asked my Dad if he could put me to work. Dad said, "Go ahead. He's full of nervous energy and never sits still. Wear him out!"

As a mason's helper, you're responsible for a variety of things and one of the most important is to be on time. I had no problem getting up at sunrise, because he would be in front of the house to pick me up at 5:30 in the morning. I started my day organizing the day's work in my mind on the way to the job site. Sometimes we would have to stop at a supply store and restock for the week, and Mr. B would always grab a pack of crackers and a beer- root beer, that is. If we were pulling the trailer, we would have to load stone and other materials at the farm. The farm was his stockyard where he kept a goat, a chicken and, in my eyes, a vicious turkey. No matter how fast I ran, I couldn't outrun that bird! I don't like turkeys, except the third Thursday in November.

A stone mason must be precise in measurements, application, texture, and consistency. I learned quickly to listen to instruction, as he would say "look here" when speaking to me and look me directly in the eye. I assured him I understood. In the three summers I worked for Mr. B, I became skilled at managing my time and learned to get ahead and stay ahead, because as he would say, "you can't afford to get behind". This job taught me to pay attention to details and be consistent in everything I do. These virtues would stay with me throughout my career as a salesman.

~~~~

CHAPTER 2

The Wreck of 1987

THE WRECK OF 1987

After being a Breadman for seven years, I went to work for a cake company. All I sold was snack cakes: cakes of different sizes, shapes, and colors. What started out as a good move would almost end my career and my life in less than seven months on the job. My previous route on the bread truck encompassed about 10 miles daily while this new one averaged 200. Tuesdays and Thursdays were longer distances and often in areas where there was little to no population, except for the occasional cow or goat.

August 1987 was a turning point that nearly took my life and left me with too many injuries to mention.

The day started overcast and gray with a light, almost mist-like rain, but much later the area would be flooded. My truck was a short wheelbase box truck with long racks inside that contained trays of boxed bakery products like chocolate, powdered, coconut, and cinnamon mini doughnuts and other goodies like cinnamon rolls, fruit filled pies, apple streusel cakes, and an occasional chocolate cupcake. Little would I know that the morning of the light rain and overcast skies would turn my/our world upside down and all the doughnuts on top of me.

I was shifting from 3rd to 4th gear when the truck took a sudden left exit off the road, down twenty-five feet of an embankment, through a farm fence, over brush and landed on its right side. When I came to my senses, I realized I was on the ground framed by the right exit door of the truck, covered in doughnuts. I heard a humming sound from inside the truck and realized it was my makeshift fan mounted on top of the engine access lid. I tried to reach the ignition with my right hand, but my bicep was lacerated and bleeding profusely. Then I attempted to move my left arm and realized my forearm was underneath my hip and broken. Somehow, I managed to lift myself up from the doughnuts and dirt to turn off the switch.

It took a minute or two to decide what I had to do, so I pushed the windshield out of my way and rolled onto the ground. I tried to stand but fell, not knowing I had fractured the tips of my vertebrae, later discovered to be C-5, 6, and 7. Damage in this area can often leave someone paralyzed, so it's no surprise I had trouble standing up.

I crawled up the red clay, through the brush to the wet, busy highway. As I looked behind me, down the embankment to the wrecked truck, it came to me that this was bad. REAL bad! Traffic was passing a bleeding, wet, muddy man on the highway when as best as I can recall, a man in a truck stopped and lay me down on the side of the road and used his bright orange hunting vest to mark where I was.

Until I arrived at the local hospital, the minutes on the highway in the pouring rain are vague. I sure would like to thank that guy in the truck who stopped to help me. The events of that day would shake me to my core. I almost died. Somehow, I managed to recover from my injuries, and a new career soon began.

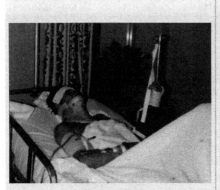

Charlie in Forrest
General Hospital

Charlie in Forrest General Hospital the day after the accident. He had surgery to remove glass from his head and face, to repair the gash in his right arm and repair the broken left elbow. The broken vertebrae were collared for stabilization.
Thankfully, he doesn't remember much about that day.

Just before 1990, I walked into a local automobile dealership to apply for a job. My wife knew the owner, so I really hoped that would help my chances of getting hired. I started training the next day with two others. And the day after that, only two of us came back. I was determined to start a new career and be as successful as my skills would take me. I was a bit naïve to start with, especially regarding commissioned sales. I had come from a career as a route salesman with a guarantee plus commission. The car business would prove to be a different animal.

In this new world I would need to use many, if not all, of the traits and virtues invested in me from Mr. B. His investment in me would pay dividends in the future, but it would take some time to reap the rewards. My career as a salesman would take me to places I never would have been able to visit, and introduce me to people I would have never had the joy and opportunity to meet. I am forever grateful for their trust to help them, their children and grandchildren. And after 30 years, there are many who still contact me to ask my opinion or advice.

Here is my advice to anyone who endeavors to sell anything. Don't lie. Never make promises you can't keep. Apologize for making mistakes because you'll rarely get second chances. Keep your intentions focused on people. Be consistent in behavior, conduct, and relationships.

I've learned how to listen, listen, listen. Why? Because there just might be something bigger going on that will, in time, change who you are and make you better and more effective at who you are, not what you do. I believe everything that happens in life has a reason and purpose. How could that 15-year-old kid, who started out as a stonemason's helper and a grocery store clerk, grow into a student minister, breadman and car salesman who would arrive at a greater purpose in something other than what I did?

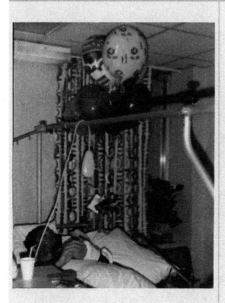

Charlie in Forrest General Hospital two days after the wreck. He had surgery to repair the broken left elbow and stich up the gashed right arm.
The wounds in the back of his head and on his eyelid from the glass were being medicated, as were the burns on his back that he suffered from the heat of the engine.

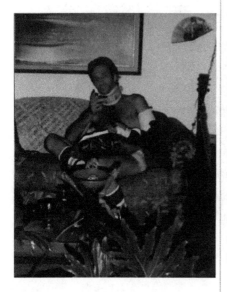

A few days after being released from the hospital, he was resting at home.

There wasn't much that could be done for the broken vertebrae in his neck, so he was in a collar for some time after. Charlie kept his sense of humor, even though it was quite painful and challenging to get up and down the stairs of the house.

~~~~~

SHERRI'S RECOLLECTION OF 1987...

In 1987, he was critically injured in a work truck accident. He was driving a route through small towns for Dolly Madison Cake Company, towns that were far apart on two-lane highways.

In the pouring rain, the truck failed, slid across the oncoming lane and turned end over end down into a ravine. When he came to from the impact, he was in the grass, covered in the metal racks and products.

There were shards of glass in his skull and his eyelid, and his back was burned from the engine. His left arm was broken at the elbow and his right arm was almost severed from the deep gash. We believe that God had His hand on this because, somehow, he was able to climb up the incline, through the briars and bushes to the edge of the highway where he fell in the rain and prayed for help. Because of the rain, cars blew past him, lying there, bleeding and muddy. Finally, a stranger saw him and stopped to cover him with his orange hunting vest and call 9-1-1. The small-town hospital ER in Prentiss did the best they could before being told to transfer him to Forrest General Hospital in Hattiesburg.

At the time, I was a reporter for the local NBC affiliate and was on assignment somewhere when my news director called. I raced to the local ambulance station where my good friend Danny was on duty. I sat next to him in dispatch listening to the EMTs describe the injuries and the situation. I prayed hard for anything good in that news, but the words 'broken neck' really floored me! It was a vertebrae fracture and, thankfully, the medical staff was able to stabilize him for the ride to Hattiesburg. That was a long, tedious surgery and several days in the hospital. But at no time was there ever a sign of any brain tumors or other cancers. I know that God's hand was all over this wreck and Charlie's recovery.

As for me, I had a job, and it kept me busy enough that I didn't hover or wring my hands in despair over the near-death experience he had. I worked for some great people who gave me leeway with hours so I could be at home more. After all, we had kids in school and Charlie was facing a long road of recovery. I think this was my first genuine experience as a 'caregiver'. We figured that time would heal him, he would find another job, and things would be smooth as silk from then on. Boy, was that wrong.

I guess you don't take life too seriously until you have stared death in the face. That's the time you call out to God! And He will answer, because He's always been there, waiting for you.

Sometimes the weight is too heavy, and I just can't pray. Crazy, right? When that happens, I send a text to one of my church sisters and they will call and pray over me. During terrible, unexpected news, it's okay to cry out to the Lord, "Why, God? Why me?"

It's okay to question the hard stuff, but remember, no matter what you're walking through, He is right there with you.

Deuteronomy 31:8 *"It is the LORD who goes before you. He will be with you; he will not leave you or forsake you. Do not fear or be dismayed."*

We were very involved in our church activities and that was such a blessing. Our church family came to us on all levels and supported us during Charlie's recovery. I don't know how we could have gotten through this time without the people who called, visited, brought food and even took our children to church when we couldn't. There was a time in our lives that we weren't in a church at all. Looking back, it was not a good time for any of us. When people tell me they are struggling in the aftermath of an accident, or catastrophic illness or even a divorce, my first question is always "do you have a church family?"

A decade later, we would face yet another major hurdle, Charlie tells it from his perspective.

~~~~~

CHAPTER 3

Ten Years Later- The First Brain Tumor

IN OCTOBER '97, I WOKE UP WITH THE WORST HEADACHE EVER!

My head hurt so bad that I basically lost vision. Our son Joshua was 16, so he drove me to the hospital. In the late 90s, the emergency room was pretty simple. I was in a bed surrounded by curtains. The first thing they did for me was a shot of some kind, probably a steroid, to ease the pain followed by what seemed like hours of waiting. I've been told distraction was provided by my family, who were busy trying to blow up gloves on their heads.

I can't say I remember that at all, but I do remember a nurse came in to collect a blood sample, which raised my suspicions. What have they found? It probably was just a few minutes later I decided I'd been there long enough, so I got up to pull the curtain and almost bumped into the doctor.

"You're not going anywhere! We found a suspicious spot on the last scan of your brain. We aren't certain what it is, but I'm recommending admission."

Dr. Michael Fromke, Neurosurgeon, sure knew his stuff. Here was a brain surgeon who described the biopsy procedure like a painter describing every stroke of his brush on the canvas. He explained that the machine that he was going to use could accurately pinpoint the spot within the diameter of a ballpoint pen. I was mesmerized and ready to proceed.

After the "drilling a hole in my head" affair was over, we were told that the spot, not actually a tumor, was nothing more than a harmless, benign astrocyte. We really had no idea what any of this meant. All I can remember is we were told to have annual MRI's.

We never thought to ask why. We had no idea to ask where this diagnosis was leading. We were completely naïve and had no tools with which to research.

We purchased our very first home computer in 1998 and suddenly, the world wide web was at our fingertips. However, except for setting up email and playing spider solitaire, we didn't really have a clue how to search for information on brain tumors.

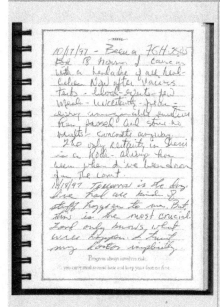

His journal: 10/17/97
Been at FGH for 18 hours. I came in with a headache of all headaches. Now after various tests—blood—events—few meals—uncertainty—fear—every imaginable emotion has passed. And still no results—concrete anyway. The only certainty is Sherri is a rock— always has been when I've been down for the count.

In less than 30 days, the surgery will happen.

His journal: 11/18/97
Tomorrow is the day. I've had all kinds of stuff happen to me, but this is the most crucial. Lord only knows what will happen. I trust my doctor implicitly. I also trust my life in the hands of God as I always have. Probably not as well as I should most of the time, but in matters like this it brings you around to your senses. Makes you realize what matters most— family, children, friends; and what doesn't really matter at all. At this moment I certainly pray that I'll be all right. If the prognosis comes out not good, then we'll move forward from there. The only way I know how to deal with things is to proceed straight ahead. There is no need or future in sitting still and not doing anything.

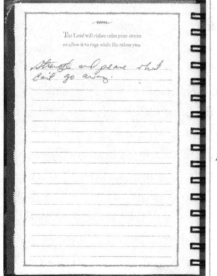

In order to be positive and have the promise of tomorrow, I have to be looking ahead.

Where there is no tomorrow, there is no hope; where there is no hope, there is no future. Hope is the piece of rock I cling to.

This is my hope: Sherri will be strong and resilient. She has been all that any man could want in a wife. Never in 1000 years could I wish for another. I love her more than anyone in this life. She is my soulmate, my past, my today, my tomorrow and future

. With her I have a strength and peace that won't go away.

SHERRI'S RECOLLECTION...

I was so thankful Josh was home from school that day and drove Charlie to the hospital. They called me at work. I met them there and not too long after that more family members showed up, so it was a full room. We kept each other entertained trying to blow up gloves with our noses. The staff said they were running the usual tests, but we honestly weren't expecting anything but a sinus infection or migraine. Imagine our surprise when the doctor said they found something of concern on the CT scan of his brain. Dr. Michael Fromke was the neurosurgeon in Hattiesburg at the time. He was honest and up front but also very relaxed and spoke to us in everyday language.

For me, the shock of hearing 'brain tumor' was devastating. My usual attitude is 'get the facts, take over, make a plan, get it done.' At the time, we had custody of our 20-month- old granddaughter. When the neurosurgeon explained there would be some side effects from the biopsy, I knew I would not be able to care for Charlie, take care of a toddler AND work full time. As much as it hurt, we decided to take her back to my daughter in Tennessee for the time being. Dear Lord, I can't remember ever crying for eight straight hours, but I did that day, and most of the trip back.

Between that biopsy procedure and 2008, we basically forgot about anything in the brain. Charlie continued to have annual MRIs up until 2005, then just stopped going. We were in full-time work mode and raising an elementary school kid. In 1999, I got a call to co-host a morning show, so back I went into country radio. Charlie was still working at Petro Automotive and loving it. He has always been honest and loyal to his customers.

In May of 2000, we lost my grandmother, my rock, my heart. And then in October that same year, we lost Charlie's Dad. That was so hard. They say you shouldn't make any big decisions when you're grieving, but in November, we packed up our home and moved across town in less than a week to our first new 'new' home.

Joshua graduated in May 2001, and three months later, Hanna started kindergarten, so we started over. Looking back now, there were no big medical emergencies in those years to speak of. There were symptoms, though, that we should have paid more attention to while they happened.

At least five times in two years, Charlie suffered what he categorized as sinus infections, eye issues, earaches, facial pain, and headaches. Taken as symptoms, it's easy to see why a family practice doctor might be inclined to treat each thing with a separate prescription. What didn't click to us was that these were also symptomatic of brain tumors, and Charlie's probably could have been detected at a much earlier stage than when it was finally discovered in December 2008.

The symptoms of a GBM are masked in everyday ailments, until it reaches such a stage that it really affects your ability to see, to stand up straight, and even causes seizures.

Pay attention to the small things, and when they start adding up, it is your right to ask for an x-ray at the very least.

~~~~~

CHAPTER 4

The Devastation of 2008

A BIRTH AND A NEAR-DEATH

SHERRI'S RECOLLECTION OF DECEMBER 2008.... FROM CLARKSDALE TO VICKSBURG TO HATTIESBURG.

Monday Dec. 8, 2008 — Sun. Dec. 13th.

We spent the weekend in Clarksdale celebrating the birth of Lexi Claire, our second granddaughter on Friday Dec. 5th at 10:54pm. Ben and Alicia are going to be great parents!

Charlie wasn't feeling well enough to drive, there or back. On Sunday when we detoured through Vicksburg, it was obvious he was having real trouble. The headaches and blurry vision had progressed to the point of interfering with everyday functions. On Monday he was too dizzy to work but insisted on driving himself to the emergency room where the CAT scan revealed that a brain tumor had basically 'blown up'.

This is how the week of highs and lows started. Our family was now facing a real fight to keep Charlie alive and healthy.

We got to the hospital in Clarksdale early that Saturday morning, but Alicia's labor was slow going. We spent most of the day wandering the halls and eating snacks from vending machines. At one point, while we were camped out on the floor of the wing, Charlie was so sick that I wanted to flag a doctor to check him right then. He refused to let me do that, choosing instead to suffer the intense pain of a migraine that, of course, we later discovered, was not just a headache.

There were signs something was seriously wrong in the two years leading up this event, although we didn't add them all up. You would think the most common would be headaches and blurred vision, and you would be right. But he also had severe earaches, described as 'fluid' and balance issues. He saw his family practice doctor several times complaining of a sinus infection and was prescribed medications to treat the symptoms.

Please do NOT self-diagnose! Please do NOT tell your doctor what you think is wrong. Instead, ASK for some tests-even weird tests that don't sound like normal protocol. We truly believe that having a common x-ray would have shown the progression of the tumor long before it grew to almost the size of an egg.

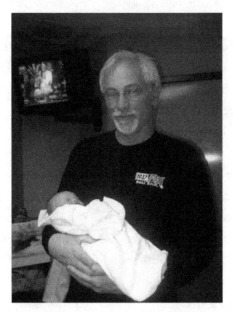

Poppy holding newborn Lexi Clair! He was so
happy to meet the newest grandbaby, but you
could see in his eyes, he wasn't well.

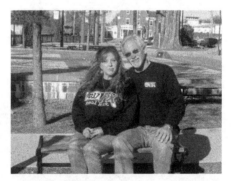

The following day, Sunday, on our way home,
we stopped at Vicksburg Riverfront Park.
While we sat on the bench in the cold, Charlie
said the words on the history marker were
moving. I drove us the rest of the way home.

The ER trip was a Monday. Surgery was set for Wednesday. Although he doesn't remember, he did have visitors in between. Several friends and co-workers stopped by just to share a word of encouragement or a promise to be there no matter what. It's so much more important than you realize to have people—just your people—who don't think twice about coming to see you or bring food or pocket change. We had always been the ones who showed up to bring snacks or prayer, so when our time came, friends were fast to return the favor. I am probably the worst, though, at letting any emotion show or even asking for help. My nature is to be brave and 'in-charge' rather than let someone else do for me.

Going through this devastating moment in time was hard. Of course, it's difficult for the patient. My goodness, there's something in their brain trying to kill them! But for the significant other, well, all we want to do is fix it. And I couldn't fix it.

My emotional state zipped back and forth from being on task to hyperventilating to reassuring him to wondering if I was going to die. And as I look back now, I can say it's okay to feel ALL that. There are days now, in the quiet times between doctor visits and scans, that I will catch my breath and tears will threaten to fall. But then I can say out loud, "Jesus, take the wheel!" because I don't have the power, but He does. Please remember that. He expects us to call to Him. That's what God wants to do for us.

As the wife, caregiver and support system, on the outside I kept it under control. Everything got done, everybody got where they were supposed to go. When the tumor was removed, the treatment began, and we were so blessed to have my parents to help as well as our church family.

But at the same time Charlie was having radiation treatments, I was taking care of my birth father, who was battling esophageal cancer. I would go into work at 5:30am, do the morning show until 10am, take care of work duties and then, most days, leave by noon to drive Dad to the VA two hours away in Jackson or take something to his house. He spent weeks in the hospital and still managed to get free time with us at home.

Somewhere in that February to April window, my adult daughter was admitted to the hospital for treatment of lung issues related to her previous drug addiction. I did the best I could to help her, to at least be there, but I'm afraid I fell short.

Lord only knows how many miles I logged between hospitals, clinics, work and home. I was grateful for my job—so grateful! For those four hours every day, I left all the sickness and worry outside. Keep in mind we had a child in school. Hanna had just turned 13 and middle school is hard enough without both parents running all over the earth and an extremely sick great grandfather she had only just met. She was nurtured by her school counselor, who prayed over her, and she was accepted into the family of 'band'. That sure did help her stay grounded.

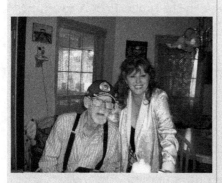

Sherri's birth father 'Johnny' on Christmas morning at our house. He was in the late stages of esophageal cancer and was struggling to swallow anything. He had to go back to the VA hospital in Jackson later that day because of the pain.

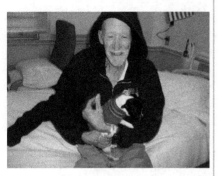

Johnny in his room at the VA hospital, the last time he got to hold his Baby dog and the ONLY thing that brought that smile. He passed away just a few days before his 87th birthday in February.

Charlie had some really ugly side effects from the Temodar, and the radiation burnt his poor head. I tried to be gentle and supportive, assuring him this was just a temporary speed bump in our lives. On the outside I was calm and under control. On the inside I was borderline hysterical. There were times I had to pull over on the highway and just cry my face off, sometimes only a couple of minutes. Then I would suck it up, clean my face and drive on.

I did all the things you would expect one to do when faced with something this difficult. I begged. I bargained with God. I promised I would go to church more. ANYTHING to save my husband. I had to stay strong for him, though, and my Dad and our kids.

Looking back, I should have had someone I could let go with. I've never really done that, not even now. Anytime he was in the hospital, someone would volunteer to stay with him for a couple of hours so I could go home and shower and love my dog. It also gave me that time to fall apart, even if it was only for that short time. I am being very raw and honest when I say it's OKAY to do that—to just fall apart. But don't do it in public and try your best not to become a puddle in front of your person. On the inside, they, too, are just screaming in fear, but they're depending on YOU to stay strong in the fight.

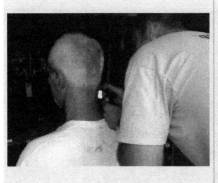

During the treatment and recovery period, our son Joshua cut Charlie's hair in anticipation of his losing some of it.

He was always good with the clippers he inherited from his great grandfather, Red Morgan, and the inherited talent from his Italian granddad, a barber by trade.

During treatment, Charlie also thought it was a good idea to build a shop in the backyard. He wanted to have a place for all of his tools and to work on vehicles other than in our garage.

With some help from his brother Chris, our neighbor Jim and the boys, it was a nice project that has provided some much needed funds at times over the years.

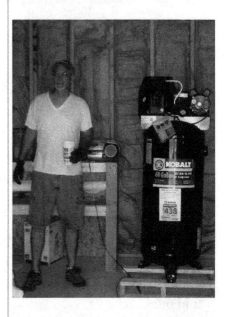

CHARLIE'S VIEW: DECEMBER 8, 2008—THE DAY THAT CHANGED OUR LIVES.

We had enjoyed a very busy but gratifying weekend. My daughter Alicia and son-in-law Ben became parents to Lexi Claire. I was driving home from Clarksdale and, when we got to Vicksburg, I had to hand the wheel to Sherri because of a headache and problems managing lanes and distance on the road. That was a long Sunday drive.

When I got to the dealership Monday morning, I walked some 100 steps to my office to sit down and begin my To Do list. The headache was still there! I never thought the next decision would always echo in my mind. I felt like my blood pressure was extremely high and my heart was pounding so loud my ears were aching.

I started back to the front door and said to the receptionist, "I don't feel right, something is really wrong."

"You don't look so good, Charlie! You better be careful," she replied.

When I arrived at Forrest General ER, I told them I had no idea what was wrong, but I felt like my head was going to explode. As I turned around and looked back toward the door, Dr. John Nelson was arriving. Here he comes, the head of the ER department, late for work on a Monday!

I said "Hey Doc. Late on a Monday? Let me guess, it had something to do with your wife's car?"

He laughed. "Yes! Now what are you here for?" I explained some of my symptoms, and he said, "It's possible it could be that tumor."

Brain Tumor? From 1997 to 1998? How could that be? The neurosurgeon back then told us we had nothing to be concerned about. The original biopsy had revealed a benign tumor the size of the point of a ballpoint pen. No way.

Questions, nothing but questions. Dr. John Nelson made things happen so fast, I don't remember Sherri arriving at the emergency room. All I remember is going in for a CT scan and (maybe) back to the ER cubicle. It wasn't too long after that I was headed to the MRI only to find just what the CT showed was a suspicious tumor. It is important to note: There were several symptoms that were evident most of the summer of '08. I was having problems with eyesight and concentration, anxiety, sinus pressure, headaches, equilibrium and even my temperament. Sherri can probably add to the list.

For the remainder of Monday, December 8, 2008, I have zero memory. I don't remember a thing after having the MRI. I may or may not have had visitors on Tuesday, but if so, the day is vague and foggy. By Wednesday the 10th, I woke up and felt so much better. In fact, I decided to take a walk down the hall of the neuro floor. Approaching the nurses' station, I was 'about faced' right back to where I had come from. Wednesday and Thursday passed and we had no idea what we were in for. But we were about to find out.

Psalm 63: O God, you are my God; earnestly I seek you; my soul thirsts for you; my flesh faints for you, as in a dry and weary land where there is no water. 2 So I have looked upon you in the sanctuary, beholding your power and glory. 3 Because your stead-fast love is better than life, my lips will praise you. 4 So I will bless you as long as I live; in your name I will lift up my hands. 5 My soul will be satisfied as with fat and rich food, and my mouth will praise you with joyful lips, 6 when I remember you upon my bed, and meditate on you in the watches of the night; 7 for you have been my help, and in the shadow of your wings I will sing for joy. 8 My soul clings to you; your right hand upholds me.

On the 12th the neurosurgeon came in either late afternoon or early evening and gave us the news. No one, especially us, was prepared to hear the word 'cancer'. CANCER! We were told years ago the tumor was benign, and now it's malignant? For a few minutes (that felt like hours) we sat speechless.

The doctor asked, "Have you ever seen the Grand Canyon?"

Grand Canyon? What are you talking about? No, we haven't. And suddenly it hit us! This is not good, not good at all. I asked, "How bad is it?" His answer, "The worst it could be. Pathology graded the tumor as a Glioblastoma Multiforme IV."

Cancer comes at you like a freight train. It comes in various types and grades. These were things we had no idea about, and certainly were not prepared to absorb any of the specifics and language that comes with the diagnosis. When the doctor gave us the news I asked, "What do we do now?" What is the plan? Whatever I have to do, let's get it going!" By midnight, the radiologist and oncologist visited. We spoke briefly, but there was a temperament in the room that left us with a very uneasy feeling.

The average survival rate for GBM patients isn't very encouraging. Only about 25 out of 100 survive after 12-15 months. After discovering the low rate of survival, it would be a GIANT hurdle if I passed the one-year mark. This was going to be the biggest challenge of my life!

It is so much better to be proactive than reactive when it comes to a cancer diagnosis. I wasn't given a cancer owners' manual. The internet became my best friend and worst enemy. Which brings me to this well-known advice: don't believe everything you read because not EVERYTHING on the internet is 100% true. There were searches done that would make the most unemotional person break into wailing and uncontrollable weeping. Again, nothing prepares you for this! It is cancer and it is out to kill you.

1 Peter 5:6 Humble yourselves, therefore, under the mighty hand of God so that at the proper time he may exalt you, 7 casting all your anxieties on him, because he cares for you. 8 Be sober-minded; be watchful. Your adversary the devil prowls around like a roaring lion, seeking someone to devour. 9 Resist him, firm in your faith, knowing that the same kinds of suffering are being experienced by your brotherhood throughout the world. 10 And after you have suffered a little while, the God of all grace, who has called you to his eternal glory in Christ, will himself restore, confirm, strengthen, and establish you. 11 To him be the dominion forever and ever. Amen.

~~~~~

CHAPTER 5

The Journals of 2008-2009

Here I sit - dog in my lap - watching a re-run of House that I've seen 5 times, and staring at a mostly naked Christmas tree. I can't find the spirit - can't even fake it enough to pretend Christmas is 15 days away. Every day it gets harder to stay in the moment - to allow myself to feel - anything. On the outside, I should be happy - I'm expected to be something - but now I can't find it. Don't care - about the holidays or the house. Having a lot of trouble putting forth any effort - have to make myself call family - Forcing myself to get up and go to work- force myself to walk - all the while knowing what should be done. I don't want to do this 'surgery'- don't want to be down for even a day let alone several. Angry because I'm being torn between being here at home and my need for theatre.-

So depressed about no money to even try to buy presents and even if there was, I can't say I would feel any better about it all.
I don't understand this underlying simmering anger in me. There are little points of happy every day but not enough to keep me here 'in the moment'. I feel so fake about lots of things. Like my faith. I can't even make myself - LET myself - feel things. I can't be like Charlie - go to a place where he is - and it seems I can't make myself feel guilty about not feeling. Just don't care... some days it's hard to not keep driving - to just give up on all of it. Some days I would like to stop moving altogether - But I feel the need to take care of all the details and make sure everything was organized first.
And I wonder when or if I'll feel better- Sherri

Charlie's Journals of 2008-2009

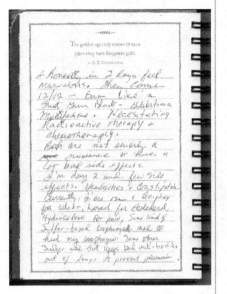

I honestly in 2 days felt marvelous. Then came 12/12 – Bam - like a shotgun blast - Glioblastoma Multiforme. Causing radioactive therapy & chemotherapy.

Both are not severely a nuisance or have a lot of bad side effects. I'm day 2 and few side effects. Headaches and constipation. Currently I'm on Rx for ulcer, Rx for cholesterol, hydrocodone for pain, some kind of Sulphur-based med to heal my esophagus. Some other med that keeps bad antibodies out of lungs to prevent pneumonia.

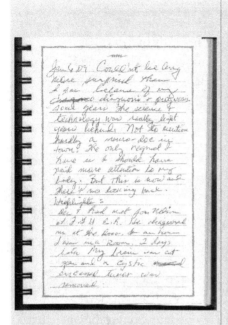

Jan. 6, 09 - couldn't be any more surprised than I am because of my diagnosis and prognosis. Some years the science & technology was really light years behind, not to mention, hardly a neuro-doc in town. The only regret I have is I should have paid more attention to my body. But this is now and there is no looking back.

Highlights: Dec. 8 I had met Jon Nelson at FGH ER. He diagnosed me at the door. In an hour, I was in a room. 2 days later my brain was cut open and a cystic-encased tumor was removed.

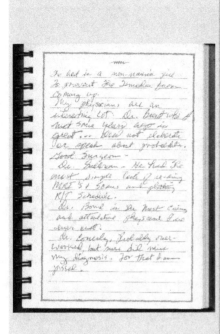

The best is a non-nausea pill to prevent the Temodar from coming up. My physicians are an interesting lot. Dr. Brent who I met some years ago is great...does not elaborate or speak about probabilities. Good surgeon.

Dr. Salloum - He had the most simple task of reading MRI's & scans and plotting R/T schedule.

Dr. Bond is the most caring and attentive physician I've ever met.

Dr. Conerly, probably overworked, but sure did miss my diagnosis. For that I am pissed.

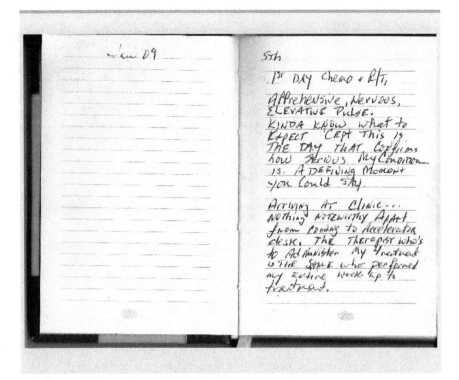

Jan. 5th- 1st day chemo & R/T.

Apprehensive, nervous, elevated pulse. Kinda know what to expect this is the day that confirms how serious my condition is. A defining moment you could say.

Arriving at clinic... nothing noteworthy apart from coming to accelerator desk. The therapist who's [sic] to administer my treatment is the same who performed my routine work-up to treatment.

8th- Really good day. No big hi's (sic) no big lows. More or less just trying to relearn my body's changes as I enjoy therapy. Trying to understand the changes come with some relativity. I'll be worse later before I get better. Did notice I lost 4lbs. Hope the trend slows down, concerned about my stomach & intestines, however.

Psychologically makes me eat less & less. (PM) went to bathroom, thought I'd solve my digestive problem. Let's just say it's too horrible to describe. I do have a newfound appreciation for babies with colic though.

I pray I never go through that again. If the cancer don't kill me, my digestive track will. 9th- Sherri's b-day. This is a very nice day- simply put, one of the best by far. Gotta repeat, went to the bathroom without fainting- enough of that! Radiation was a snap and chemo went without a hitch. So far so good, almost done with 7 days chemo, 5 of R/T. 10th- Hanna's B-day. Trying to install radio in Envoy, didn't work. Already have a perfectly [good] 5 year old CD player. Pissed off now, will resolve in the morning. Have noticed by 3pm really have a downturn in strength & energy. Managed to lay down and by 5:15 felt good.

11th- Watched football last nite, same thing today. Nothing new to report. Feel like I've been sick forever. This is such a slow process.

12th- The start of 2nd week of treatment. Most of the time I wouldn't even know I've had brain surgery; however, it has been a month and I do feel better. No dizziness, tiredness, weakness, everything feels so normal it's scary. Getting bored with nightly routine.

13th- couldn't sleep much last night, body & mind's adjustment to no medication. Yes, I'm not on anything at all. That's great. But I of hope I can get some sleep. Can't shut my mind off! Good day, got the Mustang running- really do not want to sell it. Means more to me (Sherri) than most know.

14th- didn't sleep last night again. Felt terribly washed out yesterday. Had no energy.

Most of my day has been spent trying to sleep. But no hope. Think I'll be fine after today. Radiology was fine, becoming somewhat boring. Noticed we're radiating the same area in the same sequence every day. I take this is good, they're isolating the site where the tumor was. I'm still not sure how the Temodar works. Need to ask or read.

15th- a much better day. Got some sleep finally, Probably gonna feel run out some of the time. Spent most of the day resting. Need to organize my days to include more physically active things.

16th- pretty good day overall. Today marks close to 30 more til I'm done. Had a real defining moment this evening. Broke down in front of Sherri.

21st- Gonna check into changing my schedule. Noticed after radiation my throat gets really dry & tight. Eases up later but might make chemo easier if it was earlier in the day. 2 more days till I'm halfway done - sure was nice to have Sherri home today.

22nd- Thursday - can't wait til this week is over.

23rd- Had Dr. Bond appt. this morning - got really good news- Blood work was great. Head back later for radiation. Going to eat Mexican tonite - reward & celebrating.

This was a bad night on chemo - intestinal ache was rough.

24th- Good most of the day. Noticed after taking Bactrim I had that weird fainting feeling again. I used to call panic spells. Believe I'm probably allergic to Bactrim.

Notice if I lay on right side, stomach pain is less, even after taking chemo. Need to control the bathroom function and not strain anymore. I'm becoming increasingly concerned about these spells. Hope this is not a shadow of the future. Then again if medicine can control it, I'd be willing to do what's needed.

25th- really good Sunday. I like weekends better than weekdays.

26th- Had a meeting with Dr. Salloum, he said I could take Temodar any time of day. Date of completion will be Feb. 17th. 27th- Nothing new, spent the day getting car ready for paint. 28th- Painted car. Finally this close to being done.

29th- Danny has been my ride, don't want to take any chances at this stage. Had an afternoon spasm on my left side, just above abdomen, felt shock up to my neck.

30th- did some research on my left side - seems the spleen and pancreas are there - to me, feels like my spleen is swollen.

Decided to lay on my right side, seems this reduced the left-side pain. Propping my legs up for a few helps. Overall, Friday was really good. I'm worried so deeply about the stress that's on Sherri when it comes to Josh & Chivonne.

31st- 16 more chemo days, 13 more radiation!

1st- Superbowl Sunday. So far, so good, took chemo around 2:00, no problem. 2nd- Had a moment in radiation - hope it's just anxiety and not something else.

3rd- Heart skipped a beat at some position in radiation, but not as bad as yesterday.~~

Journaling is a great way to let your feelings and thoughts and concerns just flow.

Prayer journaling is also good because you can write out the prayers and petitions to God even if you can't speak the words out loud. You should be journaling your life anyway, but if you get a diagnosis of cancer, go right away and buy a couple of three subject spiral notebooks. WRITE IT ALL DOWN. While you are documenting your feelings and fears and prayers, remember there are others you know who have been where you are or are going through it now. Pray for them, too. Believe it or not, there are many folks out there who have cancer but prefer to keep the struggle to themselves! In the final chapter of this book are resources to help you find solid information for your journey.

1 Timothy 2 First of all, then, I urge that supplications, prayers, intercessions, and thanksgivings be made for all people, 2 for kings and all who are in high positions, that we may lead a peaceful and quiet life, godly and dignified in every way. 3 This is good, and it is pleasing in the sight of God our Savior, 4 who desires all people to be saved and to come to the knowledge of the truth. 5 For there is one God, and there is one mediator between God and men, the man[a] Christ Jesus, 6 who gave himself as a ransom for all, which is the testimony given at the proper time.

CHAPTER 6

The Healing Prayer

During the treatment for the GBM, there were dozens of calls and visits. One such call was from a family friend, a church member, who spoke healing and called out to God while on the phone. Emmett Wayne Creel will never know the effect his prayer had that day. But God knows. And we truly believe that He heard that plea and that declaration from Emmett Wayne for Charlie's healing. Months and even years later, doctors still want to question the original finding, because "nobody lives this long" with that brain tumor. As Christians, we accept the fact that The Lord heals us from our afflictions—one way or the other. If not here in this lifetime, surely when we get to Heaven.

~~~~~

CHAPTER 7

A Brand New Thing

—AND NOT IN A GOOD WAY

CHARLIE RECALLS 2015-

As early as seven years after the initial tumor resection, I began to have seizures. The hospital stay was lengthy. The stress on Sherri was beyond my comprehension at the time because I have no recollection of the events. When released from the hospital, I was on three medications to control my brain and prevent seizures. One of the medications was $700.00 for a 30-day supply. It didn't take too long for us to work out a solution that was affordable and functionally effective, but it was still hard to deal with at the time. The last thing I wanted was to become controlled by the medication that was necessary to prevent my seizures. Many seizure medications cause lethargy and a slowing of cognition. Lord knows I have had enough brain matter removed that the last thing I needed was to impair the leftovers!

Since I really don't have any memory of those ten days in the hospital, I will turn this chapter over to Sherri.

SHERRI ASKED "WHAT IN THE WORLD IS THIS?" JANUARY 2015

Jan. 24th - 10:30am

I was putting on make-up and getting ready for work when I heard Charlie from the other room. It was the weirdest sound, like "oh oh OH OH" and I came out of the bathroom to see what he was 'oh'ing about. He was standing in the doorway between our room and the kitchen and was kind of shaking and his eyes rolled back. I just knew it was a seizure.

Before he could fall toward the kitchen floor, I bear hugged him and managed to get him down on the carpet in our room. It took all my strength to let his head gently touch the floor. I was talking to him non-stop and trying to get to my phone to call 9-1-1.

The entire time I'm talking to the emergency dispatcher, I'm also getting dressed. He was still, breathing good but gurgling and with his eyes open. I hoped he could hear me talking to him and answering questions from the 9-1-1 operator.

The ambulance must have been close because I heard the sirens about the time I opened the garage door. Thank goodness he was already dressed, and as they loaded him on the stretcher, a good friend also pulled up in the driveway and volunteered to follow me to the hospital. After a few hours in the emergency room, they determined he had had a seizure but not a stroke. He was given the all-clear and we went home.

Jan. 25th- 12:54pm, he had another bad one.

This time he was standing up at the bar. And let me tell you, we have the most dangerous living room ever with four glass-topped tables, so I held him as tight as I could while he shook and struggled. My phone was nowhere near me but my Kindle ® was on the bar, so I reached with one hand

and flipped it open. Hitting messenger, I typed this to my daughter who I knew would see it immediately:

"help, he's falling. Call 911. Cant hold him"

She called and the ambulance got there in minutes. By that time, I had laid him down on the floor with pillows under his head. He came around and the EMT's worked on him in the ambulance in the driveway. Once we felt he was okay again, he was awake and alert enough to answer questions and I brought him back in the house.

We joked about just leaving the ambulance in the driveway for the rest of their shift.

That probably would have been a great idea because the third time he had a seizure, it was, thankfully, while he was laying down and the EMTs were standing by. There goes another $1,000 ride across town to the hospital and the emergency room. This time I wouldn't let them discharge him. I demanded they call his neurosurgeon and admit him.

He was admitted and continued to have seizures that were mostly like 'zone outs', where he would just stop talking and start to turn his head up and to the right.

Sometimes he would start saying 'oh oh oh' and the seizure would last from a minute to as long as fifteen minutes.

The doctor ordered the EEG monitor so for two days straight, he had electrodes all stuck to his head with a camera recording his movements and a monitor recording the brain waves. It was scary as hell for me. Every time he would 'go out', I would stop breathing, worried this would be the last time we had a chance to talk. I may have been on the verge of panic more with this hospitalization than any other.

Because he wasn't all there, his impulses were sudden, too. If he decided he had to go to the bathroom, he would jump out of bed and start that way, still hooked up to the leads and even a drip once or twice. It took me and a few others to contain his movements.

He developed the habit of tuning everyone out if he was eating. It was funny more than once, but our family has always found humor in hard times. I was so very grateful to have adult kids around: all three of the girls and Joshua, too. Our son-in-law Shelton was there a lot, helping to get Charlie around or keep him from leaving a couple times.

Our church family was in constant contact and our ministerial staff was there every single day praying over us. We even had the famous local Irish Catholic priest, Father Tommy Conway, come and pray over him.

Those ten days in the hospital were so hard on our family. My heart broke and I had to fight crying openly just to see Charlie in this way. It was sad and scary, and I was almost paralyzed with fear every time he had another episode, wondering for just a minute if this was the last time he would connect with me or anyone else.

I prayed almost constantly, maybe never saying 'amen' because it was a steady stream of petitions to the Lord to heal my person, the one who makes me the person I am, the other half of my heart.

Matthew 19:6 So they are no longer two but one flesh. What therefore God has joined together, let not man separate.

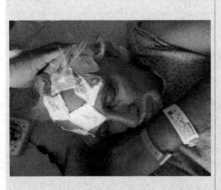

Every seizure episode would tire him out, and you could really see it in his eyes. If it was hard to watch, it was doubly hard for him to have that physical reaction on his body. The monitors stuck to his scalp were very uncomfortable.

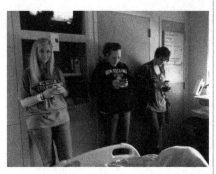

They didn't say it out loud, but you can see Alicia, Chivonne and Hanna were really scared. The three of them still managed to cut up and tease Charlie when he was 'awake'. They kept their phones in their hands, texting each other the funny things Charlie would say and egging him on to keep talking.

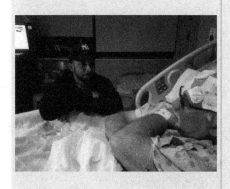

Josh would drive all the way from Picayune to Hattiesburg in the pre- dawn hours to talk to him and encourage us before he left for work, driving the hour back to Pearl River County.

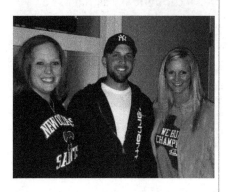

While Charlie was in the hospital, I realized our children had grown into some awesome adults.
Pictured:
Chivonne, Joshua and Alicia

A note here. Don't hide things from your kids. DO ask them to step up and help. They are waiting for some direction, and it's up to us to give them a way to feel useful during this terribly stressful time.

Sadly, over the years, I have become pretty good at sleeping in the chair-beds in hospital rooms. I have it down to a science now and even bring my sleeping bag for some extra comfort. But you still don't sleep soundly. If he even moaned or coughed, I was up. It seems we can't just go in for a day or two. It's been ten days every time. My feet hurt all the time from the walks down the hall to the elevator, then through the halls to the parking garage. But I had to get out for an hour or two every day to go home, see my dog and cry in the shower. I can't remember if I went to work at all that week, but I do remember my co-workers calling and coming to visit. I was so grateful for a work family that truly cared about us and wanted to help any way they could.

I'm going to be really honest here. I was scared to death. I begged and pleaded with God, forgetting that I could claim victory. I forgot we HAD that victory back in 2008! All I could see was us not making it to our 40th or 50th.

When he had that first seizure, I thought I was having a heart attack. My chest literally hurt from the pounding and it was all I could do to not throw up in my car on the way to the hospital. I needed to call people but I didn't want to call anyone. I needed someone to stand with me but I said, no, I'm good, thanks. In the past I had gone to work to escape the hospital, but this time, I was afraid to walk down the hall for coffee.

Christian singer/ songwriter Matthew West released a song in November 2020 called 'Truth Be Told', and it covers what I was feeling at the time:

Lie number one, you're supposed to have it all together. And when they ask how you're doing, just smile and tell them, never better.

Lie number two, everybody's life is perfect except yours, so keep your messes and your wounds and your secrets safe with you behind closed doors.

Truth be told, the truth is rarely told, I say I'm fine, yeah I'm fine, hey I'm fine, but I'm not- I'm broken.

And when it's out of control I say it's under control but it's not- and you know it.

I don't know why it's so hard to admit it, when being honest is the only way to fix it.

There's no failure, no fault, there's no sin you don't already know so let the truth be told. {1}

During this stay, Charlie went from 6th floor to 9th. They tried to bring him out of the seizures with a shot of Ativan which usually worked after a minute or two. However, one time, while he was in the bathroom, he had a seizure episode that lasted almost 45 minutes! They couldn't give him another shot. I was freaking out; the kids were freaking out. Even a couple of the nursing staff were at a loss. At one point, there were three nurses in that tiny hospital bathroom trying to help.

I finally put my foot down, and when that happens, I tend to get loud. "Somebody better do something RIGHT NOW!"

The charge nurse came in and said there's a team whose job it is to override everything and everyone. All I had to do was call the operator and give her a code for our room number. Less than two minutes later the door swung open. A doctor and two techs came in and told everyone else to get out. He demanded some answers about the reason the seizure was allowed to go on that long and why a certain medicine hadn't been given.

I don't know exactly what they did or how they did it, but Charlie came out of that seizure and was able to respond. I'm not saying you should do this but if the situation is warranted, and you just can't get any satisfaction with the present treatment protocol, tell them what you want or call the operator.

As a caregiver, remember you are also the patient advocate for your loved one. You're not the doctor or nurse but they should be able to answer any questions you may have. There is a 'patient rights' document that is signed as part of HIPPA which gives you and your person the right to ask for second (and even third) opinions, to request a different set of eyes to look at the situation.

There are now 'hospitalists' on every floor. They're like family practice doctors but just for the hospital and, for the most part, it's good to have them on call to answer any questions.

For some reason, we had this one doctor who wanted to give Charlie a psych evaluation. She believed he was faking the seizures to get medication. I pretty much lost my cool at this point and told her to get out of the room! As I backed her into the hallway, my daughter holding my arm, I added that if she so much as stepped foot near his room, I would call security. She understood me then and we didn't see her for the remainder of his stay.

She wasn't the only one we had an encounter with while on that floor. Even though Charlie has a neurosurgeon who is on his case at all times, there was a call for a neurologist. The man, while excellent at his job, had the bedside manner of a crocodile. I give everyone the benefit of the doubt to start with and, because I am my husband's advocate, I have to be the one to stand up for him. Occasionally you will get a physician who just doesn't give a flying burrito what you have to say and will bark orders out right over your head and your objections.

I've been dealing with Charlie's health and brain issues since 1998, so I do have an idea of what he can and cannot take. My encounter with this particular physician played out like a scene from a soap opera.

This neurologist walked in the room, demanded some answers from the nurses there, gave some orders and walked out. He never acknowledged me at all.

I asked the nurse, "Who was that?"

RN: That's your husband's neurologist."

Me: "Wait just a minute here."

I was so shocked at his attitude it took me a minute to blink, and then I went to the nurses' station and asked where he was. They said he was already off the floor. I said, "Get him on the phone right now." He was about to experience the wrath of the redhead.

When he did call back, I left it on speaker and the conversation went something like this:

ME: "Dr. Smith, how dare you waltz into my husband's room, bark at the nurses, yell out some orders and walk out and never even speak to me. I am his WIFE and I say what does or does not happen with his treatment. You won't ever do that to me again. When, and IF, you do come back, you will speak directly to me and not him. Am I clear?"

MD: "I apologize and I will consult with you the next time I make rounds.

Me: "Thank you!"

I think the nurses actually applauded.

Again, you are the one who must stand up for the person with the brain tumors. They can't always understand the severity of the situation, or even answer questions from medical staff. So, it's up to US to be sure they get the very best care whether it's in the hospital, the cancer center or the clinic.

After a few days of the monitor, Dr. Brent came in to explain what he felt was causing the seizures. The cavity where the tumor had been in 2008 was developing scar tissue and it was blocking the communication between left and right brain. It wasn't termed a regrowth but scarring. We took comfort in that because we needed to take comfort where we could find it. They started him on anti-seizure medications, heavy duty at first and tapered off in the days ahead.

Ten days in Forrest General. Ten. Long. Days. Finally, we got the news that he could go home with the medications in place. Our kids were so happy, our church family was happy, and I was so exhausted from it all, I just wanted to sleep in our own bed with my husband.

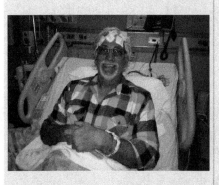

Jan. 31st- put on a happy face! Not sure if he was 'all there' when we took this photo.

Feb. 1, 2015: Super Bowl Sunday... spent in Forrest General Hospital. The whole family was in the room. We had a spread like it was going to feed 20 people. If I remember right, we even had a crockpot full of Rotel ® cheese dip, a tray of sandwiches and cakes. Everybody was trying not to be too loud. We didn't want to get kicked out, and the nurses kept sneaking in for snacks. Charlie was just along for the ride. About the time the game was supposed to kick off at 5:30, the satellite system in the hospital went out. So there we sat—staring at a blank screen. All that food, all those folks, and nothing to watch. I'm sure the kids can recall more of that day, but since we didn't get to watch it when it was live, we voted to watch a replay a few days after he got home.

Charlie said he didn't even remember that Sunday anyway so it was all brand new to him.

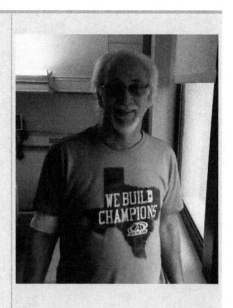

Feb. 2nd- ready to get out and go home!
Nothing like that feeling when you're packed and ready to be discharged.

We thanked God for bringing us through this trial and prayed for good health and many more years. Thankfully, he doesn't remember much at all of those days, but our kids certainly do. We wouldn't have gotten through those days if not for our kids, my parents and our awesome church family at Petal Harvey Baptist.

If you don't have a church, find one. You don't have to go it alone. There are people whose purpose is to hold others up in their time of need. At the end of this book, there are some references for you to call and connect with if you need assistance or an advocate.

Sherri's Journal-

1/28/15 My daughters tell me I need to write the book that Charlie suggested as he came out of another seizure... "Yes, I'm a pissant, but I'm YOUR pissant!" Yes, he is my pissant.

Moved to 6th floor – neuro - where we were after the brain tumor. The staff here are well versed in this brain activity. He cried earlier—so overwhelmed by having our kids here. So proud of the adults they've become. All he asks is to get out of here with all the sense he came in with.

Thursday 1/29/15 Had a good night's sleep—lost a couple of EEG leads overnight but we hope it will all go away today. Josh came in a little before 6am— had a nice chat and left for work. Five minutes later, Charlie had an episode start while...

...brushing his teeth, lasted about an hour. Brother Jason (Wade) stopped by to visit and pray with us.

It crossed my mind in the middle of all this that I haven't seen a brush or shower in two days. I need to get out of this building, but I'm scared to death to be gone. He told me this morning that he knew all along this day would come—when his brain would cause problems. I am in almost constant prayer. I must sound more like I'm begging than claiming—because we are due at least 40 more years.

It's been easier in the past to take over the household duties—pay bills, take out the trash, do laundry. I can't do anything now except ache. We are so much 'one' person that when he has a seizure, I feel like I can't breathe, and I'm unable to really focus. I wonder if his symptoms are becoming mine, too?!

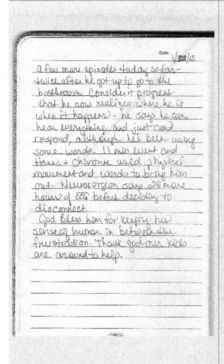

A few more episodes today so far. Twice after he got up to go to the bathroom.

Consider it progress that he now realizes where he is when it happens. He says he can hear everything and just can't respond, although he's been using some words. Eleven minute event and Hanna and Chivonne used physical movement and words to bring him out.

Neurosurgeon says 24 more hours of EEG before deciding to disconnect. God bless him for keeping his sense of humor in between the frustration. Thank God our kids are around to help.

Every time he had an 'episode', he reacted differently. Sometimes he would just stop in mid-sentence and stare off into space for a minute. Other times he would make sounds and sit straight up in the bed. A few times he even started singing a little, so Hanna would sing along and use that to bring him out of the seizure slowly. Our kids all had different ways of dealing with his seizures, but it was hard on all of them.

We thought the episodes of 2015 would be the last time we had to see the inside of a hospital, but we were SO wrong...

CHAPTER 8

2019 Tries to Bring us Down... again

March, April and May of 2019 could have and, in some spots, should have killed us. March was just crazy with the hospital stays. On April 14th my mother died unexpectedly and then in May it was more visits to the ER and the neurosurgeon's office.

Monday, March 11, 2019, at 4:30am. I guess I don't sleep as soundly as I used to because he can make any sound out of the ordinary and I'm wide awake with a hand on his shoulder. I heard the 'Oh oh oh' before the bed started to shake. I jumped out of bed, hit the lights and ran to his side to be sure he wasn't falling off the bed. It was a violent seizure. It scared me bad this time, but I kept talking to him.

"Charlie, it's okay. Hang on, you'll be okay. Just breathe." (Was I telling him or myself that?)

When he started to slow the shaking, I grabbed my phone and hit 9-1-1 as I started to find a tee shirt and some jeans, all the while talking to him. His breathing was labored, his eyes weren't really focused and he was sweating.

DISPATCH: "9-1-1- what is your emergency?"

Me: "My husband has had a grand mal seizure. He is a brain cancer patient and this seizure was pretty violent. I need paramedics fast, please."

D: "The fire department and ambulance are on the way, ma'am. Is he stable right now?"

Me: "Yes, for the moment. He's still on the bed."

D: "Is that him breathing?"

Me: "Yes."

You could hear him rattle inside his throat and chest following the seizure. He was trying to focus on me, and I was talking to him all the while. I could hear the sirens coming closer. We are less than a mile from the fire station and they tend to get here first.

"Hey, baby, I'm here. You're okay. Help is coming. You're all right now. Just hang on."

I disconnected from the dispatcher, let the firemen in the house and took a quick second to find some shoes and my keys. I felt like I was reliving the incident of 2015 when I moved my car out of the garage to allow for the gurney. It was a flurry of movement and questions about the seizure as they talked to him. The paramedic asked Charlie to roll over to his right, to the edge of the bed, but he wasn't able. He said he felt too heavy and had no strength, even though his mind kept telling him to do it. It took two people to pull him off the bed onto the gurney using the sheet.

It was déjà vu all over again as I sped behind the ambulance to Forrest General Hospital. I could see through the back window that they were installing the IV and he was talking a little. But somewhere during the trip, he had another seizure and because of the restraints, he thought his arm might have been injured.

That was another long Monday filled with scans and tests and covering work and calling family. The initial MRI showed something on the resection site, but results were inconclusive.

Dr. Brent, his neurosurgeon back on the case, ordered the EEG monitors again so they could figure out exactly what was causing the seizures.

By Friday, March 15th, Dr. Brent came in to talk with us about the results and the plan to do surgery again. It was too early to tell what the 'matter' was on the site, but he was planning to back in the same way as before to remove it. The surgery was set for Tuesday.

That Saturday we asked our attorney to come to the hospital and let us record the legal stuff. Charlie had to sign the HIPAA form so I could have full access to his records and he had to answer some questions and sign the will. In the last chapter of this book, we will go deeper into these actions so you have a heads up. {2}

Sunday, March 17th we had a mini family reunion bedside. Our son Josh and daughter- in-law Shelley brought granddaughter Mila. Our daughter Chivonne and Hanna were there and Alicia brought Lexi. My mother and step-dad were also in the room. Our daughter-in-law is an excellent stylist and Shelley gave Charlie a good shampoo to get the EEG pad adhesive out and a nice haircut in advance of the operation. We shared food, and Charlie drifted in and out the whole time. He says now, as before, he doesn't remember much of the ten days. It was also Joshua's birthday—an Italian kid born on St. Patrick's Day! How cool is that for his ancestry? Being the baby brother, the girls treated him to a birthday supper at a local Chinese restaurant.

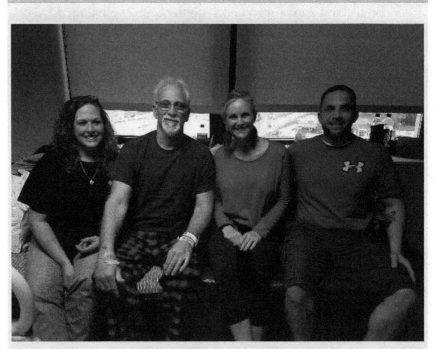

Chivonne, Charlie, Alicia and Joshua

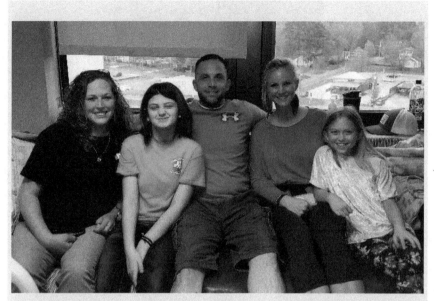

Chivonne, granddaughter Mila, Joshua, Alicia and granddaughter Lexi

Monday, March 18th We hadn't slept much because the room air conditioner had stuck at 55. We were frozen. We told the night shift folks. They called maintenance. By 4:40, we were too cold to stay in the room so we walked down the hall and found a gurney stuck under some cabinets. We sat there, wrapped in blankets and each other, and dozed for half an hour.

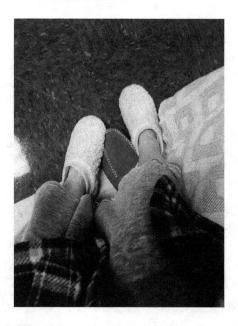

Back in the room, we watched yet another sunrise through the hospital window. The promise of a new day— the time when prayer feels most powerful.

In the almost 40 years of our marriage, there have only been a few times I have taken off my wedding band, but this was the first time I've worn his ring on my chain while he went back under the knife. Maybe I was worried that he wouldn't be there to wear it much longer and I needed it to be close to my heart.

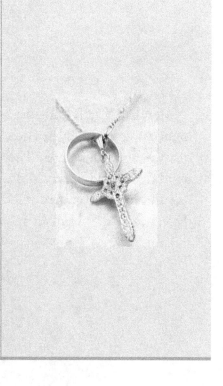

We are so blessed and fortunate to have a church family that isn't afraid to pray for us by name! That Sunday evening, my cell phone rang and it showed as Bro. Dustie Dunn, our pastor. I put him on speaker for everyone in the room to hear, and the congregation prayed for Charlie during the church service. That is the authentic way to minister to your people, and God has shown us that so many times.

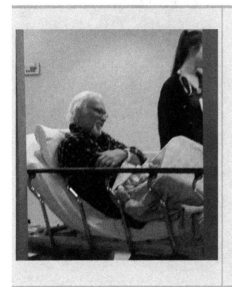

March 11, 2019
Getting wheeled down to the imaging department for yet another MRI. We have joked that because he's had so many scans, chances are by the time he's 80, he might glow in the dark. When you feel like you're on the hamster wheel of medical tests, it helps to lighten the mood sometime.

March 14, 2019
Still in Forrest General Hospital in Hattiesburg. This isn't the first time he's had the EEG monitors hooked up. It measures the electrical impulses of the brain, and hopefully, gives the neurosurgeon some answers about what could be causing the seizures. The sticky pads and electrodes are uncomfortable, and certainly don't make for a good sleep.

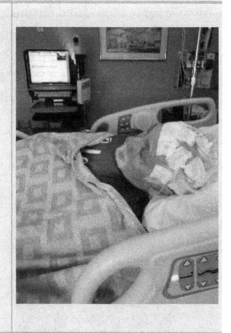

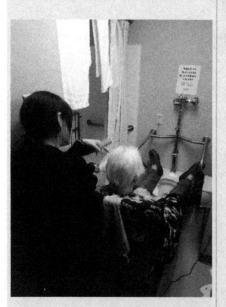

March 17, 2019
You just make it work. That's the attitude we all have when it comes to taking care of Charlie. Our daughter in law Shelley is an excellent stylist and she was more than happy to give him a nice haircut before surgery the following morning. Of course, the only place suitable for this was the hospital bathroom! His hair looked really nice even though we knew the next day there would be a mess in it.

March 19, 2019
Just back in the room from the surgery. He had a bad reaction to the anesthesia and before he got completely into the room, he was throwing up, which in turn, caused stress to the staples on the site. The nurses were really fast and had him medicated and cleaned up.

The sleep after surgery is usually good, but he was in so much pain this time. The gauze turban didn't want to stay in place and the craniotomy site was exposed. Dr. Brent made sure it was changed within hours.

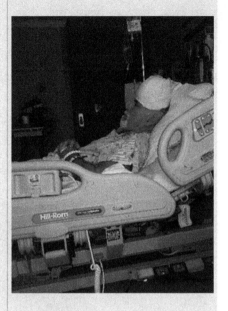

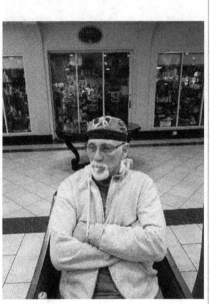

March 21, 2019
We could only stand to be enclosed in the four walls for so long before we decided to make a daring escape.

Patients, especially neuro patients, are not supposed to leave the floor.

We casually strolled down the hall, found a wheelchair near the transport elevator, and just floated down to the first floor. He wanted to see outside from the lobby where the piano sits. We spent a little time in the hospital chapel, too.

I truly believe we have the best neurosurgeon in the state, maybe the Southeast, on Charlie's case. He is so easygoing and quiet that we have nicknamed him 'The Ninja'. But bring up an automobile—ANY car at all—and he and Charlie will talk a solid 30 minutes about the merits of the engines and on and on. Dr. Ron Brent loves what he does, so much so that after he did one of the craniotomies, he texted me a picture of the 'brain hole'. Our kids begged to see it, so of course, he had to show them in the hospital room.

March 22, 2019
Finally getting ready to be discharged and that's when Charlie discovered his glasses didn't sit right because of the staples near his ear. Dr. Brent's solution? Remove the arm and just get by with the one on the left. He even carried a tiny tool set to do it, like a surgeon would. As a parting gift, Dr. Brent handed us the bag with the tools and the right arm of Charlie's glasses.

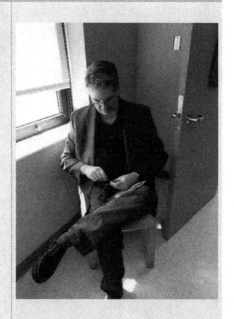

On day 11 of this stay, we made it home and spent some time with the kids and grands and prayed for some real rest. We got away from town with a trip to the coast and to Picayune to see granddaughter Mila's archery meet. Little did we know that just three weeks later, we would lose my mother suddenly after a brain bleed.

That Saturday, Mother was good. We talked, visited for a bit and everything seemed okay. Around 8ish, my step-dad Danny called and said "Wendy fell out of her chair. I called the ambulance." We raced up the road to their house as they were loading her into the ambulance. She was talking fine. In the emergency room, we all chatted about what the next meal would be and, somehow, she had grabbed the blue nail polish on the way out and wanted to be sure we would finish painting her toenails the next day. The neurologist told us she had a significant brain bleed and that they would admit her to ICU for the night to see if they could fix it with medication. There were hugs and goodbyes all around and we all left, promising to come back for breakfast. At 1am, my cell rang and it was the ICU nurse telling us mother had coded and was on a ventilator. If I thought I had moved like The Flash when Charlie had a seizure, I was a blur getting up and dressed and calling my step-dad. That was a painful call to make. We picked him up in the darkness, turned on the emergency flashers and were at the hospital in less than 15 minutes. By 5am, most of our family was in the waiting room, taking turns going in to see her. When it became clear she wasn't going to recover, they allowed all of us time to say our good-byes.

The service for Wendy Gorsuch Richardson was held April 18th at Petal Harvey Baptist Church. Our hospitality ministry prepared a meal in the fellowship hall for afterwards, a true Southern tradition, with all the best comfort foods. My uncles were both there, the middle one from El Paso and the baby brother who lived across town. It was a very hard weekend, for sure. We were thankful that my mom had planned out and paid for her funeral and burial plot years earlier, although, thank goodness, the olive green casket she had chosen in the early 80's was no longer in production. She was laid to rest in a gorgeous rose gold. We are all sure she would have approved.

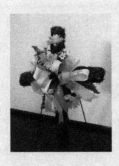

April 18th
We had the funeral service for Miss Wendy at Petal Harvey Baptist Church.

Friday May 3rd
We attended our community Relay for Life event, where Charlie was among those survivors honored. We purchased a luminaria in memory of mother.

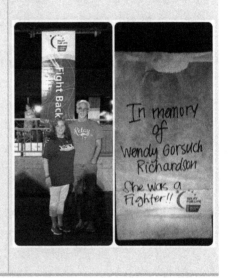

Saturday, May 4th, we had a family reunion with the Clarks (my cousins). It was a great gathering with wonderful food, but it had been a very long day. We were lying in bed watching SNL only because Adam Sandler was hosting and there was a LOT of laughter. {3} That's when he felt something wet on his forehead and on closer inspection in the light, realized something was dripping from one of the holes where a stitch had been. We freaked out and thought, holy cow it's spinal fluid! Off to the ER we went. That was a crazy all-nighter in the emergency room.

In the exam room, I had to exert some serious authority to keep them from taking unnecessary tests like an EKG (why???). I finally had to threaten one nurse to keep them out until the on-call neurosurgeon arrived.

He looked over everything, never really made a definitive call on what it was and opted for staples to close it up. In the event it WAS some sort of brain leakage, there could be no anesthesia applied locally so the staples went in POP POP (so far, so good) and the third one went POW and he almost jumped off the table. By the time we finished up all the checkout stuff, the sun was coming up on Sunday morning.

By Tuesday night, the leak had returned and Charlie complained of a headache and neck pain. According to the doctors, these are signs of meningitis. Back to the ER but it was packed! So many people were just on beds or chairs lining the halls. Because of his possibility of infection, we were placed in a tiny little room across from the nurse's station in the emergency room. It was only big enough for a chair and the bed and the bed had to be turned a little for a nurse to come in.

After a few tests, a tech opened the door wearing a gown and mask, hung a hazmat placard on the door and shut it. This was the SAME nurse that had been in and out of the room for two hours before someone finally figured out it might really be meningitis!

Our kids had been in the room most of the evening, too, and we just thought it was dumb. We were also told there were no empty rooms, but later heard there was a nursing shortage so they could only put patients in so many rooms.

It was the next morning before he got moved to a room for IV antibiotics to start after the procedure to install the central line into his heart. After everything was under control, he was released Saturday, May 11th. Home Health came Sunday and showed us how to administer the medication safely.

Thank the good Lord we haven't had anything new happen since May 2019 and he even got to ring the bell at the Cancer Center to signify he was DONE with treatment!

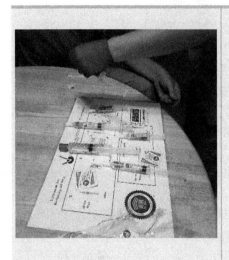

May 12th
The Home Health nurse demonstrated the medicine. We were a little apprehensive about giving the antibiotics at first.

May 17th
We had to get away. An hour drive later, we were on the beach getting sunshine therapy. That was followed by a healthy dose of Bar-B-Q shrimp.

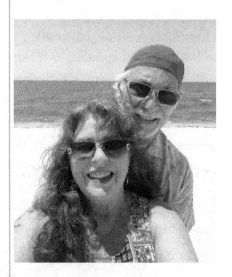

THIS IS HOW CHARLIE REMEMBERS MARCH 2019...

March 2019 was a date that surpassed December 2008. I woke up around 4:30am in full blown seizure. The most memorable thing about that morning is that I was fully aware of what was going on. While I have no recollection of ten days of seizureville in 2015, March 2019 is as vivid as if you were watching it on DVD.

That morning everything sounded muffled, but my wife's voice was clear and had an echo to it. She kept saying my name and assuring me that the EMT was on the way and to focus (as best I could) on her voice and STAY with her! I could hear my own guttural voice. It reminds me of how someone could have a seizure and be accused of sounding like an animal or even a demon.

When the EMTs arrived, I was asked to roll over on my right side, I tried so hard, but my body would not do what my brain wanted to do. I felt impaled to the bed and as hard as I tried, I could not get off my back. The EMT asked me to roll over several times, and then decided to move me by the sheet from the bed. After being rolled into the ambulance, I don't have a single memory of the trip or any additional seizure.

The next few days were about to remind us how sudden life can change. If I thought 2008 was a turning point, 2019 would become the hopeful last. Even after 15 months (July 2020) the video replays itself, at least once a week. It serves as a reminder of just how far we've come. I take some solace in the fact that I KNOW what someone who has seizures encounters.

We arrived home after brain surgery that removed another tumor and waited for the pathology report the following week. However, I do not recall leaving the hospital. The surgeon waited two weeks to remove sutures. Within 48 hours of removal I sprung a leak.

It was on a Saturday night, after showering, that I felt a thick fluid on my forehead just above my right eye. We were worn out from a family gathering so midnight on a

Saturday at a hospital with a 'hole in the head' wasn't a pleasant thought. Still, I had taped a piece of gauze on my head and walked into the ER announcing I have a brain leak. Ironically, there wasn't a soul in the ER except us. But that didn't matter, because I was placed in a cardiac room and, to my amazement, no one addressed why I had gauze taped to my head.

After two hours of waiting and refusing to be treated for heart issues, my wife demanded NO ONE allowed in the room except the charge nurse. She sure got their attention... well at least for a minute. The hospitalist entered the room then to inform us that he couldn't do anything about my 'hole in the head' but a neurosurgeon would be paged.

I had requested my neurosurgeon be contacted hours earlier, and apparently no one did what I wanted! To put things into perspective, we arrived at 12:30am, the neurosurgeon on-call arrived at 4:45am. His initial analysis showed no brain leakage. To be certain, he focused on the hole and asked me to cough. After coughing, he said, "Yep, we have a leak, I have good news and bad news." He informed us the good news was that he could close up the hole. The bad news was the hole could not be closed with any numbing agent. He said it would feel like a bee sting. The first two staples were bee stings, but the third one a GIANT-SIZED bee that made my eye wince and face twitch.

We saw the sunrise after spending six hours in an ER, and sleep was good, so good!

The initial report came from a local pathologist who wasn't comfortable with the results because of my lengthy history, so my neuro-oncologist referred the pathology to the University of California San Francisco. Upon the news of possible cancer cells reoccurring, we not only found strength through prayer, but were surrounded with support from our church family. The entire congregation gathered around to pray over us and ask God to bring healing and hope.

After the report came back from California, I was troubled because, I confess, I wasn't expecting a malignant report. The only reassuring news from the report was that the tumor removed wasn't a GBM, but an astrocytoma that could be treated by chemo and stereotactic radiation therapy.

As if the news wasn't enough to manage, we were about to encounter another enemy. One morning I woke with a headache at the base of my skull, chills, fever and chest sweats. I called my neurosurgeon and asked him if all these were normal, post-surgical symptoms, considering the leaky brain thing? He said, absolutely not! Go to the ER immediately and say: "meningitis". That'll get their attention." Well, off to the ER once again and wouldn't you know it must've been "Monday Madness at the ER". The line was so long that people were standing outside. I told the clerk "I have meningitis" and you would've thought the condition was as common as a cold! She ignored me and asked for my identification and nothing else.

Later in the day, after laying on a bed in the hall for 18 hours, the hospital went on lock down because there were no more beds. We found out much later that the real reason was a staff shortage. The overall complexity of this meant another hospital stay, with an infectious diseases doctor who could not provide a definitive diagnosis. Despite all the uncertainty, my neurosurgeon provided a course of treatment that took three days of high-powered IV antibiotics with an additional two weeks at home treatment via IV.

Unfortunately, we had yet to begin the chemo and radiation necessary to combat the cancer so the recovery period would be rougher, tougher, and longer. Perhaps the worst part of cancer treatment is the recovery period. It seems that after you've completed a month of treatment, the last ten days to two weeks is the toughest. The aftereffects on your body and mind have a lingering wear and tear. What's worse is the uncertainty about whether the treatment was successful, and what's just around the corner.

We want to take a break from our story and share some words from a friend whose experience with a GBM tumor did not have the outcome they prayed for.

CHAPTER 9

You are not fighting this battle alone!

The survivors are few, the losses are great. This is the account from one family whose Mother was moving in a positive direction, only to have a sudden turn for the worst possible outcome. Renee Stringer was diagnosed with a glioblastoma multiforme in January 2019. This is the account written by one of her daughters...

I remember like yesterday. I was at a friend's house and my sister called me. She said something is wrong with mom, you need to come to my house. When I got there, they said that she was having some tingling in her extremities and she would start salivating a lot. She had been earlier that day for an MRI. Her family practice doctor got the results and had set up an appointment with a Neurospinal specialist, saying, "There's a spot on the scan." But she was vague.

We kind of thought mom was having a stroke. Her episodes (tingling and salivating) came more and more often within the next hour. My sister and I called her doctor and then our Dad, who was in Texas. After consulting with them both, we decided we needed to take her to The University of Mississippi Medical Center emergency room. We were in the waiting room all night and finally got her taken back. We gave them her MRI disk to review and after some time, the ER doctor came to us and said, "Well it looks like a Glioblastoma."

We had no idea what he was talking about. I remember looking at mom and my sister Jessica and then back to the doctor and asking "So, is that, like, cancer?"

He very matter-of-factly said, "Yes, it is a very aggressive brain cancer." Those words cut like a knife!

That moment would change our lives forever.

We called my dad back in Texas but did not tell him what was going on per mom's request. We just told him, "You need to get on the first flight home." It was around 3am when they started admitting Mom and 5am before we ever got in the room. We were exhausted and completely defeated at that point. Here we were thinking we had come for a possible stroke and were hit like a ton of bricks and waiting to have to tell our Dad that his soulmate and wife of 30+ years had a very aggressive brain tumor.

The next morning Dad flew in and was there before we met with Doctors. When they came in, we asked the Neurosurgeon exactly what the treatment plan was for Glioblastoma. He kept saying, "Oh, we don't know for sure if that's what it is, but we are going to remove it." We were aggravated by the fact one doctor was saying it was a GBM and the other saying they didn't know for sure. We felt like he knew it was a brain tumor but he refused to say it.

Mom was diagnosed with the brain tumor on January 16th, and seven days later had the surgery to extract it. We felt that it was bad because of the speed in which the doctors did the surgery.

Mom was a CHAMP. She had over 20 people in the waiting room and thousands more all praying for her. She came out of brain surgery and. as they wheeled her down the Neuro ICU hallway to recovery, she was waving at all of her adoring fans as she went by. The Doctor was astounded at how well she did with coming out of surgery.

The next few weeks were filled with lots of phone calls and waiting to meet with her Neuro-oncologist. During this time, we decided to try and get her in to M.D. Anderson Brain and Spine Clinic. After much persistence we succeeded! They called and said they had a cancellation and could we be in Houston the next morning. I called my dad and said pack your bags we got an appointment. My Dad, Mom, sister and I loaded in the truck and took off, not knowing what to expect.

We pulled up the next morning and were overwhelmed by the sheer size of the hospital. We were running from one end to the other getting tests done, bloodwork, meeting with social workers, multiple physicians, NP's, nurses, etc. We were all impressed that, despite the size of the facility, it ran like a well-oiled machine.

We came home with a lot on our minds. There were big decisions to make, and we were completely overwhelmed. We discussed it in detail as a family and decided mom would seek treatment in Houston so we could participate in a clinical trial. She started chemo (by pill), moved to Houston for eight weeks of radiation, and every two weeks she did an immunotherapy drip as part of the clinical trial. Her team was Dr. Barbara O'Brian, Emily Nurse Practitioner, and Edmund the clinical trial nurse. They were awesome and kept us up to date with messaging through the app.

Our family and friends took shifts going to stay a week at a time with Mom so Dad could work some and she would be able to have some normalcy in such an abnormal time. It was hard for her to be away from her elderly parents and her five grandkids she ran with constantly before she got sick. The radiation was so harsh! It was hard to watch. She suffered the side-effects and even became forgetful. It was painful for us to see the strong woman who was the glue for our family become so vulnerable.

Once she got back to Mississippi from Houston, Mom still had to go every two weeks for immunotherapy drips. The entire time she had to go back and forth she was on treatment, and all doctors were completely amazed at how well she was maintaining.

However, we noticed her memory and cognitive skills were deteriorating and when we went back in September for a checkup, we were told that the tumor had continued growing.

This whole time, we were being told, "This looks like radiation flares, not new tumor growth." Honestly, this pissed me off because I felt if they had tried treatment sooner, she might have had a fighting chance! In October, they scheduled another surgery to try and remove the tumor. Once again Dad, Mom, Jessica, and I loaded up with several other family members and made our way to Houston. Mom did her pre-op check ins, blood work, etc. and we all went for a good dinner before the long day ahead. We had just gotten in our rooms and laid down when the phone rang.

You know that feeling you get when the phone rings late at night? It can't possibly be good news. And it wasn't. The call came from Houston and it was the surgeon, who said "Mr. Stringer, I've been looking at your wife's MRI and there is just no way I am going to be able to successfully perform this surgery."

We all cried and cried and went to bed knowing we weren't looking at a good appointment the next day. The doctor pretty much summed up what we already knew: they could continue treatment but with no guarantee. We had big decisions to make once again. Should we come home and continue treatment or put her body through the wringer traveling to Houston when we knew the treatment would be the same?

In the meantime, I had set mom up with a Medical THC clinic in Louisiana. We began THC and CBD drops under her tongue every night. After all was said and done, we honestly think this is what gave her the quality of life that she kept until the end.

Mom was tired a lot and her memory was fading but she was still the same ole Mom, NAE NAE, Nana and wife that everyone knew and loved. She never let this horrible disease get her down.

It was not until the last few months that she really began to fade. She was losing the ability to walk and do for herself. We would put her in a wheelchair and move her around and still take her to do as much as we could. We stopped all treatment and let her have the rest of her life in peace. The last two weeks were probably the hardest of the whole year. Having our kids see the strong loving Nana that had taken care of all of them not be able to talk to them anymore or eat or walk was devastating. Having to care for our mother as she faded was one of the biggest honors of our lives even as much as it killed us to watch her suffer.

This was a lot harder to type than I thought it would be. I guess I didn't realize how hard it would be to relive every detail. I am glad you are doing this and shining light on the monster that is the disease that stole our Precious Mother!

Janna Stringer, Petal MS

~~~~~

FROM SHERRI'S JOURNAL NOTES: MAY 22, 2020- MONTH THREE OF THE PANDEMIC KNOWN AS CORONAVIRUS.

It's a Friday morning and we're still in the 'stay home—stay safe' mode and so I am just doing chores. The text from my friend Wayne came out of nowhere.

Wayne-"She went downhill considerably overnight. The hospice nurse thinks she is in the final stages, on her way to confirm."

ME: "Aww man, do you have anyone else there with you? Do you need me to call the church?"

Wayne- "I've messaged the pastor. He just replied. The nurse recommends stopping food and fluid."

God, I hate those words. Like, 'okay, we puny humans can do no more for this human'. It hits me in ways I can't even describe. Like, she is my personal friend even though we never met face to face. Like, her husband is a lifelong friend, even though we were just business associates before her diagnosis. GBM brain tumors are a terrible thing to have in common. But here we are, sharing the pain and the symptoms and the hopes that it somehow, miraculously, just disappears!

But it doesn't disappear. Brain cancer is harsh and mean and doesn't let up until mercifully, you leave your poor body behind for the streets of gold. And there but for the grace of God, go I.

One part of me is hurting for my friend, because he is losing his wife. Really, he lost her before this, when the brain tumors didn't respond to treatment but the treatment wreaked havoc on the rest of her. I'm hurting for the both of them. Life is supposed to go on, to allow you to celebrate your 50th wedding anniversary, smiling over cake and being okay with the silver hair and laugh lines.

Part of me is spiraling into a small panicky thought nagging in the back of my head. "What if?" What if I have to be where he is? What if I have to be the one to make that decision, to stop food and fluid. To stand there and be gentle enough to let go. And now I'm crying for all of us.

There's the most random thunderstorm happening and for a second, I think the heavens have opened up and cried with us today. I'm sure there are millions of people around the world going through a crisis moment right now, but this is our little corner of the world that's being rocked.

I waited a bit. Sent a message back. "We are stopping what we're doing and praying for you both." And we did because right at that very moment, that's the best we can do and that's all we can do. We were so thankful she was at home, thankful that, during this quarantine time, she was not in the hospital where she might die alone. I take some comfort in that.

"Psalm 77: 16 When the waters saw you, O God, when the waters saw you, they were afraid; indeed, the deep trembled. 17 The clouds poured out water; the skies gave forth thunder; your arrows flashed on every side. 18 The crash of your thunder was in the whirlwind; your lightnings lighted up the world; the earth trembled and shook. 19 Your way was through the sea, your path through the great waters; yet your footprints were unseen. 20 You led your people like a flock by the hand of Moses and Aaron."

And in my heart I plead, Father, please take her gently, and peacefully, and give comfort to the ones left to mourn. For some time we do that, and we are sad to the deepest part of our souls in this hurt. And yet, I can find a little smile and praise because she gets to see our Savior face to face! Hold onto that. And to quote Van Zandt: Get right with the Man. {4}

~~~~~

CHAPTER 10

A Walking Miracle

IN CHARLIE'S WORDS...

I know without a doubt there is hope and help for others who are walking this path. To live a life with passion and purpose is desirous of the most precious gifts. Sometimes life comes at you like a locomotive, speeding along the rails, and you can't escape because you just didn't see or hear it coming. Then again, you're running at the speed of light and everything goes blindingly dark, so dark, you can't see your hand. Now that's awful and painful. The thought of just existing— being a survivor consumed by medication and pharmaceutical side effects? That is neither passionate nor purposeful. I consider it a gift to be a survivor. There are times it can frustrating to see others die in their fight and yet, here you are, alive and well. Sometimes unworthiness creeps in. I've heard it called survivor's guilt. I'm not sure that's accurate when peppered with a desire to fulfill a purpose.

I've been called a "Miracle Man," but I'm not 100% sure what that really means. I was healed in 2009. Does that mean that I can be un-healed? There are multiple examples of people who were healed in the Bible. I am certain they were healed, some instantly and others in a matter of moments.

Even someone like Lazarus who was raised from the dead, inevitably got sick, became old and succumbed to death.

I have had so many brushes with death that it is getting old. Well, I shouldn't rush things. But it seems like I am on my 7th life of a cat's nine. Where do we begin? Perhaps the real question is just what is going on with all this? Is there a bigger, deeper, hidden, or obvious reason?

Nothing prepares you for the news "You had something in your brain and we aren't 100% sure it's all gone." Truth be told, I was scared into surviving.

It is hard to describe the internal struggle with a deadly disease. On the one hand, you want to move on with your life and really live whatever time you have left. On the other, everything comes to a screeching halt! Your days are consumed by medications, appointments, and counting down days.

There is a tipping point. When there are more remaining days of treatment than you've already endured, you can become frustrated, tired, and more tired. Fatigue is a slow and sneaky thing.

I cannot begin to describe how tiring it was to not be able to STOP the process. To have your world turned upside down and to know your wife is unable to get a full night's sleep because she lives with the same fear, fatigue, and probably even greater worry than any one person should have to endure.

As a cancer patient, I focused more on fighting the evil trying to kill me. Throughout the first year, countless hours were spent avoiding the negative news afforded through the internet. When the survival rate is less than 10% and the leftovers from treatment and progression of the disease leave you with no quality of life—these are not fears without foundation. They are real, and as soon as you realize there is no way out of this madness and mess, you learn to deal with it.

You eat with it. Sleep with it. Sit in treatment with it. Cry with it. Scream with it. Agonize with it. Any way to avoid the mess you're in brings the realization that YOU aren't the only person experiencing this.

At times I've contemplated the reason for all this, and I guess it's natural to question your survival, not necessarily the diagnosis. Why someone gets a death sentence illness is not an unreasonable question. Early on, we asked why this could be cancer because we were told years earlier that the tumor was so small (1999) that it was benign and 'nothing to worry about'. If there is one thing to question, it's the pathology results. When you've never had this experience and walked through the trials, there's no knowledge or information that might give you the reason to question much of what is going on.

You should always be careful to surround yourself with as much correct information and knowledge as can be found. In the years since our earliest event, the information available and technological advances have brought light and hope in unimaginable ways. The speed of these advances has had a dramatic effect on mortality rates. In short, where there used to be the NO HOPE sign hanging over your head, now there is HOPE. Additionally, it's vital to avoid negative comments, and especially harmful and inaccurate internet searches.

A very real and ever-present aspect of brain cancer is the fact that at any given minute your life can change. I've lived through trying moments involving a vehicle accident, had my head cut open twice (drilled into once) and survived. But no matter what comes and goes, there is the real, and I mean REAL, part of life that reminds me that at any moment everything can change!

My brother Chris and I have discussions about life and death. It's never been an uncomfortable subject primarily because of our faith and experience. In October 2000 I had the unforgettable experience of getting a call from our dad at 5:00 AM. He was dead within the next 45 minutes. The last thing Dad said was, "I told you I wanted this to happen at my own home." Unfortunately, Dad's living arrangements were not adequate for him to die at home. When I arrived at the hospital, no one had gone into the room and changed the look on Dad's face. It remains in my memory to this day!

There are some things you just do not forget. There are things that we all wish we never had to see and do. In life we are guaranteed, as the Bible assures us, that we have an assignment with death. The order of life is this promise: There is temporary life in this body, and eternal life awaiting us with God our Father and Creator and his Son Jesus.

What a day that will be!

Death becomes a component of life, not necessarily on a daily level, but clearly it can be and always IS in the back of my mind. I see no benefit in approaching fear and uncertainty without faith and trust. I am still learning the meaning and joy of faith being the substance of things hoped for and the evidence of things not seen. The multiple times I have faced death have not been by accident. It's been from a disease that has changed me and will not go away. I do not have cancer anymore. At least that's what we believe, but having been a repeat customer with brain cancer certainly does put a different spin on it! I have no idea how I will die, but I know one day I will.

The cause of my death is not the issue. As far as I am concerned, I've had to deal with the reality of dying since this journey began. My life is not worse because of cancer, but perhaps (as contradictory as it sounds) may be better.

I have come to conclude LIFE is not about how much you can possess. It is hard and conflicting to know that I can't do a thing to STOP what happens inside my head or brain. God knows, if there was a way to spare myself worry and pain regarding the "things I cannot control" I would, but in the medical world of brain disease, too often what you are left with is not the desirable outcome for the caregiver, or the survivor.

It has to be equally as hard and more painful for Sherri to NOT be able to do anything to help save me from my brain.

I know that sounds strange, but it is very real in this recurrent condition. In her mind, I imagine the fears and worries are greater than any I could ever have. Yet, my concerns are not the same as hers. Why? Because I don't want to leave her. I don't want to leave my children!

As awful and hard as this is to state, I find it difficult to feel like being in heaven is better than living this way. But should that moment arrive, then just remember what Paul wrote to the church at Thessalonica.

I Thessalonians 4:13-14 *"Brothers and sisters, we do not want you to be uninformed regarding those who sleep (notice to the believer in dying we simply sleep) so you don't grieve like the rest of mankind, who have no hope. For we believe God will bring with Jesus those who have fallen asleep IN HIM. According to the Lord's word, those who are still alive (in this body) who are left until the coming of the Lord will not precede those who've fallen asleep."*

So, I see exactly how I will die. I will take a last breath (and we all will eventually) and sleep! Cool, right? Still there is so much to do. I am certain that there are many people who have the same struggles and trials that both of us have dealt with and need our help. They don't know what to do, what to say, how to deal with "all this", where to turn, and is there light at the end of the tunnel? Well, maybe that's what "all this" leads to?

Ecclesiastes 3:1-4 For everything there is a season, and a time for every purpose under heaven; a time to be born, and a time to die; a time to plant, and a time to pluck up that which is planted; and a time to kill, and a time to heal; a time to break down, and a time to build up; a time to weep and a time to laugh; a time to mourn, and time to dance.

I have heard these words all my life, but never truly comprehended their depth until **cancer** entered my life. As odd as that might sound, it will probably do the same to someone we know within our years on this planet.

And it truly is difficult to hear the "C" word, a life altering enemy! Throughout the years of this battle, I have had to make a conscious decision to not allow the frustration with diagnosis, the complexity of treatment(s), the difficulty, if you survive, of living with the changes that aren't always immediate, and the time it takes to become either bitter or better.

There are plenty of things that can make you bitter, angry, depressed, down, or whatever definition comes to mind when facing cancer. When we first heard the diagnosis, our initial reaction was to question the results. To question the validity of a diagnosis may not necessarily be a bad reaction, because in that moment we were like an infant entering the world. We weren't prepared to interrupt life with doctors, tests, treatments, and terms for which we had NO foundation or reference. In a very short period of time, you learn new words and a lot of initials—like MRI, CT, PET, are just a few that come to mind. The same goes for treatments accompanied with qualifying words such as protocol, clinical trials, survival rate, and Tumor Grade.

The words you NEVER want to hear but will now learn more about than all the rest are: Glioblastoma Multiforme, also known as GBM. We heard this term and had no idea what the Oncologist even meant, but we were about to get an education. When you are forced into this arena, the only thing you can see is cancer.

Aside from the possibility of dying from this disease, bitterness can become as infectious as the cancer itself. The access for information through the internet can become your best friend or biggest foe.

My first ninety days involved time off for recovery and thirty-three sessions of radiation combined with chemotherapy. At the time (2009) the treatment protocol was Temozolomide, a new word that would become synonymous with survival, better known as Temodar. The side effects of this chemo are readily available on the internet now, but in 2009 we had limited information. In order to control nausea from the chemotherapy, Zofran was the fix. While I never had nausea, there are side effects from these medications that are different for everyone. In my case, the chemo and nausea medication, and probably the radiation treatments, caused tremendous dehydration.

Notwithstanding, my intestines suffered terribly and going to the bathroom was extreme and sometimes in vain.

Some of these statements might sound familiar: "I can't do another treatment, not today!" "What happened to me?" "Was there something I could have done to prevent or recognize this sooner?" "I've become part of a new community." "God, look at all these people struggling." "When will this end?" "I just want to be normal again." "I'm going to make it!" "No way! CANCER is not going to beat me." "Where did I go?" "Time goes by so fast!" "Don't be bitter, Be Better!" "I am so tired!" "I'm just so......tired......"

Your whole life can become a noisy highway when cancer treatment takes control. There are days when it is healthy to be angry, but let the anger or frustration of what has happened go down with the setting of the sun. Finding a place where you can pull over on the fast-paced treatment highway is necessary to release the emotions that may be just below the surface or ever present.

Finding ways to calm down and catch a breath from all the changes that stress even the most patient person proved to be my saving grace, kept me focused on the treatment process, and made even the darkest of days brighter. The days, weeks, and miles will seem slow, tedious and never ending, but as soon as the half-way point is passed, an entire month or more has flown by. After a while, I noticed a change: I no longer thought about cancer every moment of every day.

I'm a student of the Bible. I love the encounters where Jesus performs healing and physical restoration to someone. One story that comes to mind was the paralytic at a pool at Bethesda. Jesus asks the guy a question: "Do you want to get well?"

There's not a single person with any kind of cancer that wouldn't love to hear that question! Maybe there's more going on in this story than meets the eye. To be brief, this paralytic wasn't the only person at the pool. In fact, everybody knew him, as he was a frequent pool patient. Problem was- he needed help, but others received help before he could make it into the pool. Imagine what it would be like to be without any hope, or help. I think the "pool guy" had become frustrated, tired, despondent, and yes, hopeless.

When the averages for brain cancer survival are so small, the mind does play tricks on you. Fatigue, frustration, and even hopelessness can become very real and, like the pool guy, a daily routine that feels endless and possibly futile. Just when it seems things are at their worst, "Do you want to get well?"

If any of this fight was easy, I don't think I would have "tuned-in" to hear the question. Another story comes to mind that is MUCH MORE meaningful and encouraging.

There was a paralytic who had many friends, probably relatives, who came to his aid when they heard Jesus was in town. They made certain he met the Savior! And I wonder, how long was this man paralyzed? Had he spent all he could to get well? Was his wife able to manage all his needs? Did he run home? What did he do for the rest of his life?

I am ever grateful for my father-in-law who went with me to my last two weeks of radiation treatments. Several years later he would depend on me to drive him to the doctor for a procedure. I was grateful to return the favor.

It might sound contradictory to say "cancer made me better." After a few days of treatment something changed inside of me. I stopped thinking about what I was going through and started looking around me. I saw suffering like never before. Maybe for the first time I ran right into the reality of what real suffering is.

While I walked into the Cancer Center, others had to be rolled in by a wheelchair. I sat and read while waiting, while another would never read or see a sunrise again. Oncology, Radiology, and Neurology facilities are full of not only suffering people, but of people like all of us who have heard "it's cancer." Is it possible, maybe even more probable, that being aware of others can make us better? I confess, it took brain cancer to open my eyes and see the real needs of others.

One of those turning points was at my job. I sold cars for 25 years. Three years after my first diagnosis, a young couple with their child came to see me in the heat of a Mississippi August. Our initial discussion concerned their current car that the a/c had stopped working. After sharing with them how difficult it must be to ride in a car with no air in August, I noticed their child was uncomfortable and pale. I was raised in the heat of South Mississippi and don't ever recall being pale from heat, only red in the face like your Italian grandmother pinched your cheeks. Before they left, they told me about their struggle to save their child and how they had spent all they had in doing so. They were simply trying to make their lives a little bit better. Instead, they made mine a lot better because I really noticed and took time to understand the reasoning. For a moment, I wanted to be the guy that could lift their worries and lower their concerns before Jesus, just like the story in the Bible. I was able to help them purchase a vehicle with cold air conditioning and they left with lighter concerns and a more reliable car.

Change is a constant and often slow process, but I was beginning to see it coming at me like a crashing wave! I started to see, really SEE the person who had a limp and thought about why they were that way instead of just seeing a limp. When I sat in a waiting room with someone who couldn't stay awake, whose eyes were dark and sunken, I realized I was doing far better than I could have ever imagined. I was "paying attention". There are moments that have brought chills and left me speechless. I felt that way after being told that I was a rare survivor.

I had completed 33 sessions of radiation and Temodar, and my doctor wanted to get a PET scan. She wanted to get a definitive scan on our progress, so off we went to have radioactive dye shot into my veins. While in the waiting room, I saw a man with an ear to ear scar. As I introduced myself, he began to smile and says, "So you're the other one." My Oncologist told me she had only one other patient who had survived a GBM for more than five years and I wasn't even at five months, so meeting him gave me encouragement and a greater hope.

Another time I was at a little country church where my brother was preaching and sharing his and his wife's story of cancer struggles and survival. She had died within the past year, and so much of what he was sharing was fresh and inspiring that after the morning service grief and death took on new meaning... and cancer too.

As we were leaving, a woman walked up to him and said, "My husband died last November from brain cancer." I believe I interrupted the conversation without considering the value that she and my brother could have had in sharing their common experience, to ask what type of brain cancer. To my surprise it was the same as mine.

Her husband had been diagnosed in 2009, a year after I was diagnosed, and had been okay for about ten years and suddenly another tumor had grown. Her story gave me goosebumps and made me feel so unbelievably blessed. If I had not gone with my brother that weekend to a little country church, I would not have met someone who was still grieving yet knew the power of life beyond the here and now. There is more to the cancer experience than treatments, and doctor's appointments. While we may not like to admit it, death is a real and present thought.

I feel as though I have only begun understanding becoming "better" after cancer. It is indeed a day-by-day life that has had its share of ups and downs. I pray daily to not become bitter while here on earth!

~~~~~

CHAPTER 11

Get Your Affairs in Order

Some hard lessons learned...

Our insurance had a high deductible, and when you have a major procedure in the last month of the year, you're about to get hit twice. There is nothing that prepares you for that shock. It's not healthy to struggle with financial and insurance issues that you have no control over. What's healthy is to focus on your struggle to beat the daylights out of the unseen killer!

If you feel like you can't make ends meet, don't be afraid to ask for some help. Don't let pride get in the way of survival for your family.

There are various places you can receive treatment and meet other specialists. Our insurance company offered to take care of us if we chose to leave Hattiesburg and seek treatment at M.D. Anderson Cancer Center in Houston, Texas. We had kids in school and Sherri's parents needed us, so between that and the financial end of things, we chose to stay home for treatment. And it was fine because we were blessed to get great care. If you have that option, talk to close friends and your trusted circle at church to get the real information on the best treatment.

Most importantly, stress about finances, bills, and job security will drown you and yours in ways never imagined. When you receive medical bills while fighting for your life it can be a bit of a downer. Surprise!! You're probably going to die before you pay it off. It almost feels comical.

In fact, do not avoid communicating with the facility that sent the statement. If you can speak to a human, they will listen to your story and consider your situation.

Furthermore, if the bill becomes something simply unmanageable, don't hesitate to speak with a supervisor. If your situation becomes desperate ask for a charity discount. The stress of bills from your treatment and trauma are not just yours, so be careful not to become overwhelmed by something you can't control.

There are so many more important things to stress over. And it's important to remember that stress is not just yours. Stress can and WILL affect your recovery. Recovery! That's a great word, right? Don't forget you just had your skull cut open, part(s) of your brain removed, very expensive screws put in to hold a "flap" in place, and the last few days are a blur. (Why do I have a flap in my head? Does it give better access in the event you need to perform some other procedure?)

The thing that bugs me/us is we were not informed of what to expect afterward. But, then again, the doctor may have provided some information prior to the surgery and unfortunately, when your brain has been looked at in ways it was never intended, you might not remember details. I am certain these days that much of my memory has vanished. I still wish I never said, "Really, I don't remember," to my wife. There are times it might be best to just roll with it. If someone doesn't know that you don't remember something, does it matter?

The definition of the word Recovery is to return to a normal state of health, mind, or strength. But realistically, the path toward it is hard, so hard. Because you are fighting cancer, a deadly enemy you can't see, nothing is NORMAL anymore. But don't worry. There's a new normal coming and you can and will make it!

When you become a cancer patient you are consumed by big words, long pharmaceutical words that require a translator, and side effects that surprise even the most attentive person. We quickly learned how to pronounce all kinds of cancers and tumors, as well as the treatments protocols.

But still, some things sneak up on you when you least expect it, and cancer treatment can hit you harder than the diagnosis. Fatigue takes on an entirely new meaning when treatment begins to take its toll on you. After a while you just get tired of being tired. In a seven-day period, you will see some days where you aren't "as tired as I was last week". Then you may have a day you can barely make it from the bed to the couch. It gets exhausting trying to make sense of all this adjustment in your "not normal" life.

If you're a highly functioning person, the battle begins when you're brought to a crawl. Some days you want to run like before...but you can't. Some days you want to work like before...but you can't. Some days you want to sleep like before...but you can't. There are MANY times you want to turn back time, but the one thing you CAN'T do is change time!

When you find yourself controlled by a disease or illness that tries to shorten your time on this planet, then time becomes either an asset or a liability. Getting your affairs 'in order' is easier said than done. When you find yourself alone in your own head, trying to make plans for when you're not here anymore, painful emotions begin to paralyze your thoughts. Pain can make it incredibly difficult, almost impossible, to get it done. You are forced to make certain arrangements for your last days, because you just didn't see this coming. No one ever does. {5}

The other side of brain cancer treatment is what you can and should do to better your chances of surviving. Don't drink alcohol. Stay away from artificial sweeteners & sugar. Eat healthy. Drink lots of water and electrolyte enriched fluids. Avoid extreme heat (especially if you've had radiation), but try to get some degree of sunlight, even if it's artificial. Surround yourself with positive people. And play music! Whatever music gets you going, get it going! Protect yourself from potential infection and other communicable illnesses. Keep your gastro-intestinal system healthy and be prepared for severe dry mouth, bad breath, esophageal pain, trouble swallowing, and intestinal pain. If brain surgery has been performed, adjusting how you sleep changes immediately, mainly because there's nothing like a horrible bed to alter your body position! As minor as it may sound, changing the way you lay in bed can be a major adjustment.

I cannot describe how much it meant to me to have an oncologist that spends time with you during your appointment without a timer. I say that because the facility waiting room was so full of patients that chairs were set out in the hall. I discovered almost immediately that there are no strangers in an oncology waiting room.

My oncologist understood the power of touch. She would walk into a room and speak with me, not about me. With a single pat on the back or touch on the shoulder, I felt calm and confident that I had her undivided attention. The difference that made in my life also had a huge impact on my outlook. That a doctor would call me on a Saturday night just to check on my progress in the final weekend of treatment will stay with me forever.

If I take a moment and review the way I've lived these past twelve years, I feel like I've been chasing myself and running

too fast. Yes, there are times when I don't give any consideration to what my overactive behavior does to my body, or what
my behavior does to my wife. I do not understand why I get so
involved in an activity that I pay zero attention to time. Could
it be a subconscious act? Do people who have stared death in
the face behave differently? Am I living like I'm dying?

It seems to me that I have (at least my family says so) been
able to do things in which I have no formal training. Somehow, I am able to simply visualize the project and get it done.
I think in time I will gain better understanding as to what has
or is happening to my brain. On the flip side of that, memory
is a worsening problem, so it's even more important to make
notes and keep records.

~~~~

More hard lessons—from the caregiver side...

I am a movie freak. I love movies and I love films that move
me and stay with me long after they have disappeared from the
public eye. In 1996, John Travolta starred in "Phenomenon" as
a man who saw a sudden bright light in the sky and then developed the ability to learn a new language and see the mechanics
to repair a car. His character learned to decipher code and had
the ability to move objects with his mind, or so he and everyone believed. Later, it is revealed that he has an inoperable brain
tumor. Hence the reason for the 'light in the sky'. I confess, that
one caused an ugly cry. {6}

The thing is, looking back, I might have understood more if
I had taken that 'phenomenon' into consideration when Charlie bought a rust-bucket on wheels and then rebuilt the whole
car! The film was fiction, but it did address a real phenomenon
in that a brain tumor can press on certain nerves and cause a
heightened sense of abilities.

Doctors will probably disagree with me, but if I had
thought more about the fact someone with zero training
in building an engine, rewiring an electrical system and

painting cars would succeed in doing that—not once but twice? Maybe I would have been more insistent that he get an MRI.

We all remember 'Debbie Downer' from Saturday Night live, right? {7} And we all have a person (or persons) like that in our lives. This person really believes they're helping you by giving the most real talk ever about your diagnosis, and they are pretty quick to tell you about poor so-and-so who died from that very same brain tumor!

It's good to have another person close to you that can run interference and ease the conversation away from dire predictions. Surround yourself with friends and family members who want to keep your hopes up, whose mission is to pray you through this big C word. If you don't have a circle of folks like that, it's perfectly fine to go to church— any church—and just ask for some prayer partners. You'd be surprised how comforting that can be.

What do you do when you don't know what to do? There are so many issues to deal with when cancer strikes. Fear for the future of treatment, logistics of being where you need to be, how to keep the information flowing with your immediate family but not broadcasting it all over social media. Add to that the stress of trying to keep a normal routine with your school age kids and with your job, plus the dirty word: insurance.

If you don't have great insurance coverage (or any insurance at all) I would advise that you do what it takes to get coverage. We were very fortunate that I had great benefits with my job, and that included the pharmacy. But we were still just floored at the cost of the treatment drugs. I can't even fathom how difficult it must be for families without insurance.

Your focus should be taking care of your person and yourself, not freaking out over whether you should pay the rent or the electric bill. A catastrophic diagnosis will throw your family dynamic into a tailspin. It's so important to keep your feet grounded in faith and be honest and upfront with your close circle of friends.

It's easy for me to look back and see a few times when I should have been more ardent with my 'suggestions' that Charlie not attempt some things that he clearly wanted to do.

When you are helping a cancer patient who is also your spouse, there's a fine line between nagging them to be careful and saying, 'okay honey, if it makes you happy'.

There have been a few times I really had to be the bad guy —and that's just a risk you have to take. It hurts my feelings to have to stop him from doing some things that could be detrimental in the future, and he gets just as frustrated with me, too.

Brain cancer makes your head hurt in so many ways. Add to that the treatment like chemo and radiation. All that trauma on the thing that operates your body is bound to cause some memory lapses and questionable motives. I don't want to be the one standing there second guessing every single thing. That's exhausting for both of us.

You need to remind yourself now and then that patience is the key to caregiver survival. There will be times your person just gets so frustrated with you being "mom" that it causes serious rifts in your relationship. If you feel that coming on, call a family member or friend to come hang out for a couple of hours and you take a drive. Let things calm down and then talk it out. Remember, they are twice as scared as you are for the days ahead and most of what they're trying to do is remain as normal as possible.

I can't find the words to explain how much it hurt me to see him so exhausted. The month would start with energy and a smile. Then came treatment. And slowly, like a battery running down, by about four days later he would get up, get coffee and get to the recliner where he stayed most of the day. Even walking to the mailbox was a chore.

Getting adequate rest and nutrition during treatment is so important. Food and water is not just necessary to live, but it becomes fuel to survive when you have cancer.

In the first days after a diagnosis of brain tumor, here's what you need to do: buy a real journal and a couple of pens you love. Unload your feelings and fears and prayers. This also helps later down the road when you get dates and places mixed up.

When talking about surgery, things you should consider first:

Don't try to plan the next five or ten years. Concentrate on today, this week and your family.

Allow yourself time to fall apart, but don't camp out there. On the flip side, don't put on a happy face and tell everyone that everything is fine, because it isn't.

Be as real with your employer as you are comfortable being. This isn't going to be a typical surgery and you won't be 100% at work again for some time. You do have rights under the FMLA.

Go to church. Seriously, go to church. If you don't have one, talk to your close friends and tell them they can do more than pray for you. They can save you a seat.

LIVE. Really enjoy each day. Love your people.

Get your affairs in order. You should have done that already, but when a possible death sentence is handed down, you must get into adult mode and handle things.

PRAY. Talk to God about everything.

~~~~~

Reality check here from Sherri

Getting your affairs in order. I don't even like to type this-
it seems so... final. It shook me to my core to hear that, but
then my adult brain took over and said, put on your big
girl pants and take care of the situation.

In the beginning, I felt like I was just scattered all over. One
minute I'm thinking we need to check the life insurance and our
funeral plots and plans, the next minute I'm making a list of the
valuables in our house. I felt like we needed a family meeting to
talk about the immediate future, but at the same time, I would
put on the smile and say, it's all under control.

Seriously though, it was NOT under control. It was just
under the surface. The best way to have your affairs in order is
to plan ahead before anything catastrophic even happens.

One of the hardest things to consider is what kind of mess
you will leave for your kids to handle if you suddenly are unable
to function or die in an accident. My mother bought cemetery
plots and paid burial insurance for decades and when she passed
away, everything was taken care of and paid for. All we had to
do was plan the service.

When you are a vibrant 20-something, that's the last thing
on your mind. But take my advice and start now to take care of
things. We finally have our insurance plans and service details
organized although we still haven't paid for the funeral. It is so
expensive! That's why when someone passes away unexpectedly, you often see a Go- Fund-Me to pay for the funeral. You
can spend hours and hours choosing your pallbearers and your
music and your slide show, but if you haven't paid for the service or the casket or even the ground where they will park your
body, then you are leaving a huge burden for your family.

The average funeral costs in the neighborhood of about
$4,000.00. The casket will be anywhere from 2-4 grand and
the 'open & close' of the gravesite is extra. Spending $5,000
on a tropical vacation sounds great, but that money could be

split with your future self to get your affairs in order. We could go into some major detail about what to expect, how to plan ahead and ways to save, but asking to sit down with someone in a funeral service office is the best place to start.

The first thing I did when I could get away from the shock of the situation was to get on my knees. It has taken a LOT of years for me to turn the prayers around. The first inclination is to ask for help- to call out to God for a miracle- as soon as possible! But the way we should pray is to Thank Him First! Thank God for this cancer diagnosis because it will make us stronger in our faith, cause us to wear the armor of God and be an example for others who are unsaved.

Sadly, not everyone knows Jesus as their personal savior and when faced with a terminal illness, they crumble and panic. In Matthew 7:7-8, *He says "Ask, and it will be given to you; seek, and you will find; knock, and it will be opened to you. For everyone who asks, receives, and he who seeks finds, and to him who knocks it will be opened."*

A.S.K. Jesus. You will be healed—whether here on earth on in heaven—you have to believe!

We have always had a big circle of friends. Quite a few we consider close (almost related) friends because these are the people you can call at 3am with a flat and they will be there to help you change it in no time and not expect anything more than a thank you and some coffee. You need friends who can take care of your dog, run your kids to school or dance class, check on your parents when you can't be there. There were times that all we needed was someone to come wash dishes or just sit on the porch and laugh a little.

My first husband and his second wife are part of our inner circle. Rick and I had only been married 3 years and we share a daughter. She has been raised by Charlie, so really, she's fortunate to have 'my two Dads'. Rick was with us when the doctor gave us the news about the original tumor. He wasn't too far away when the second one came. And through it all, he and Charlie have remained friends. Maturity lends itself to forgiving the past and being civil for the future of any relationship.

You need friends.

~~~~~

CHAPTER 12

Faith, Family, Friends
and Fight

Charlie wants you to Remember:

FAITH. There's nothing like a bad diagnosis to turn your thoughts to the subject of faith. Faith is the FIRST thing that came to my mind when the diagnosis of cancer arrived. Why? Because it is in moments of life and death that faith becomes important and primary. I don't know how someone makes this journey without faith. For me, it is just impossible to hear the word 'remission' without applying your faith in God.

The battle takes on a different perspective with FAITH. Those hours in the middle of the night when you can't sleep for worry and fear are manageable with faith. The times spent all alone, when the voices in your head make every attempt to convince you that this is IT! Punch your ticket! Pack your bags! You're done for! When faith extinguishes every doubt placed in your head, the voices are replaced with, "I am with you, I promised to never leave or forsake you." Faith speaks loudly and provides hope. I am so thankful for the GIFT of FAITH.

FAMILY: This was part of the reason we decided to have treatment and trust the local doctors and specialists. Having the support of Family around you when you're dealing with matters that you can't control puts compassion (not pity) exactly where you need it most.

My children were and continue to be affected by this disease. I have to remind myself that I am "the dad" and the possibility of me being in Heaven and not here for them is a REAL component of this journey. The good news is that they have not been left out of the discussion (well maybe a bit) because too much information can be consuming and confusing. At best, I'll be around for as long as the Lord has grace to keep me here!

Next, and more importantly, is the person who makes me the husband and man I am, Sherri. The most difficult thing for me to grasp is how she manages to maintain calm through all the stressful and frightening moments, spanning no less than 20+ years.

What makes a family so important when battling cancer? Having your strength beside you and praying for you and always keeping everyone else "in their place."

And then there is the church family. I can remember in 2009 receiving cards of encouragement sent from various churches. Some of these were from families I had some association with and others I had no idea who they were, but one thing was clear: The Church Family is definitely a vital part of a healthy and hopeful strategy for battling cancer or any disease.

FRIENDS: When you find yourself alone and needing someone to talk to, there is nothing like having a friend to help bear your burden. Friends can bring perspective, relief, consolation, even when prayer doesn't seem to remedy your unrest. Perhaps a friend is an answer to prayer? It is true, when you're down and troubled and need a helping hand, you've got a friend! {8}

FIGHT: The strongest of warriors can be brought to their knees by a deadly disease. Cancer does not care. It doesn't see a warrior, a fighter, or the power of a thousand prayer soldiers. It is out to KILL you. You are in for the fight of your life.

Literally, fighting for your very existence. This is not a game. You do not get a practice session. You do not get a "do-over." You get the ring announcer: "In this corner is YOU and in this corner is CANCER!" Here are the rules: Fight! The last man standing is declared the victor!

I remember a co-worker who had less than 50% of heart function, who was stubborn to a fault. As you can imagine, there is another side to the trait. You would think a guy who just had his chest opened and his heart partially repaired, would be practical and cautious, right? But he just wasn't that kind of person. When he died, he was still working 60+ hours a week, smoking like there was no tomorrow, practically living so fast and furious the only way to survive was to either burn out or crash into the wall!

Why do survivors live the way we live? You'd think after being given a diagnosis that was so shattering and troubling, that caution and care would be the rule. But we're not all the same, and every person has their own way of "dealing with it." As for myself, I can say without hesitation that caution and care were put aside...not that I was dumb or ignorant of the fact that I could die from cancer. But what good is trying to overcome something that you can't see if you're just going to stay locked up at home and hide?

Regarding my own way of "dealing with it", as soon as I had completed my first session of radiation and chemo, I made a decision (after conferring with Sherri and Hanna) to build a shop. They both responded with, "Really? Isn't that a waste of money? You're recovering from cancer treatment, and you want a shop?" Over the years, the shop has been my refuge and sometimes my source of income.

In retrospect, I'm thankful my two girls supported me through that time even though, until now, they had no idea that I put every sheet of roofing sheathing on the thing! I wanted desperately to attack life and this disease with abandon. I have been brought back to my senses several times and had to apologize for some foolishness and folly, yet I do not regret one moment.

~~~~~

WHERE ARE WE NOW?

Certainly not in remission! Apparently, we will never be considered free of cancer in the brain. It's not all-consuming, but it is ever-present when you live and die every 60-90 days. This is the protocol for brain tumor patients- to have regular MRIs and follow-up appointments with oncology for as long as you live or until something new suddenly appears.

Much of what I have encountered during this season in our life has brought a new awareness of my own personality. I can be frustratingly stubborn, as Sherri can testify. To be honest, I think it is a strength. It may be the one trait that keeps me unwavering in my goals and undaunted by all the games your mind will play on you. As mentioned many times, nobody gives you an owner's manual for cancer, much less the deadliest brain cancer there is. So, being stubborn is a positive for me and will prove itself through the fire!

~~~~~

CHAPTER 13

That Year of the Pandemic

JANUARY 2020—THE BEGINNING OF A RECORD YEAR OF INSANITY

SHERRI writes: January 14, 2020,- I got laid off from my job with iHeart Radio. Zero notice, just 'sign here, clean out your desk', after 20 years. The shock was something that I can't even find words to describe. We had 14 days to find new insurance or continue to pay (large money) for the company coverage.

This is where the panic set in. Charlie was being referred to the Neurosurgery Department at the University of Alabama Medical Center at Birmingham. If my insurance was going to pay for that MRI and tumor board follow up, we had to rush it. So, on the 29th, Charlie's brother Chris drove us to UAB for the all-day appointment. Unfortunately, Chris has a lot of experience with UAB as his wife had had multiple surgeries for tongue cancer in eight years. She passed away in November of 2019.

The follow-up appointment with his local neuro-oncologist was a mixed bag of opinions. The neurosurgeon and the tumor board at UAB agreed there was a 'spot' on the resection site, but there was no agreement on whether it was a reoccurrence of cancer or a radiation scar. Back to the 60-day routine of MRIs to monitor it and for us to push it aside for seven weeks and worry for the seven days before the MRI.

In March 2020, the Corona Virus began to affect Americans. The nationwide 'stay home' order was given so we did just that. Except for Sunday dinners, it was just the two of us, which provided time to catch up on projects, start writing this book (and another) and really have a second honeymoon. He still has the appointments to follow up after MRI's but more than once, it's been via tele-conference. We really miss our church family, though, and it has caused us to draw closer to each other in our prayer walk.

Matthew 15:28 Then Jesus answered her, "O woman, great is your faith! Be it done for you as you desire." And her daughter was healed instantly.

Whatever time you have left on earth, make it count! Don't worry about the things over which you have no control, things like politics and the price of bread. Put down the screens and put up the faces of those you love because one day you (or they) will be gone and you will be left with memories.

Matthew 6:34 "Therefore do not be anxious about tomorrow, for tomorrow will be anxious for itself. Sufficient for the day is its own trouble.

Great advice! Open yourself up to new friends. Don't be afraid to let down your guard and be real with folks. Chances are pretty good that they are also going through a trial and need that connection. Be present in the moment! And here's a novel thought—how about you use that electronic thingy in your hand to actually talk to another person?

Carole King wrote:

When you're down and troubled, and you need some love and care, and nothing, nothing is going right.

Close your eyes and think of me, and soon I will be there, to brighten up even your darkest night.

You just call out my name, and you now wherever I am, I'll come running, to see you again.

Winter, Spring, Summer or Fall, all you have to do is call and I'll be there... You've got a friend. {8}

From both of us, this word of encouragement: get your heart right with God. Talk to your kids, your spouse, your parents. Get right with the Man upstairs.

Leaving is hard.

Leaving your family behind questioning where your soul is spending eternity is the worst.

Isaiah 12:2: "Behold, God is my salvation; I will trust, and will not be afraid; for the LORD GOD is my strength and my song, and he has become my salvation."

Be blessed in your journey, In His Service,
Charlie and Sherri Marengo

Email comments & questions to charliemarengo@gmail.com and reach out at www.broomclosetstudios.net

Some verses to get you started looking deeper into The Word

<u>Acts 4:1-2</u> Stretch out your hand to heal and perform signs and wonders through the name of your holy servant Jesus." After they prayed, the place where they were meeting was shaken. And they were all filled with the Holy Spirit and spoke the word of God boldly. ~

Isaiah 38:16-17
"You restored me to health and let me live. Surely it was for my benefit that I suffered such anguish. In your love you kept me from the pit of destruction; you have put all my sins behind your back." ~

Isaiah 57:18-19
"I have seen their ways, but I will heal them; I will guide them and restore comfort to Israel's mourners, creating praise on their lips. Peace, peace, to those far and near," says the LORD. "And I will heal them." ~

Jeremiah 33:6
"Nevertheless, I will bring health and healing to it; I will heal my people and will let them enjoy abundant peace and security." ~

3 John 1:2
"Dear friend, I pray that you may enjoy good health and that all may go well with you, even as your soul is getting along well." ~

Philippians 4:19
"And my God will meet all your needs according to the riches of his glory in Christ Jesus." ~

Unless otherwise noted, all verses of the Word are from a New King James Version of the Bible.

{1} "Truth Be Told" written and recorded by Matthew West, album "Brand New" 2020

{2} www.fivewishes.org

{3} SNL with host Adam Sandler, air date May 4, 2019 NBC Television

{4} "Help Somebody" written by Kip Raines and Jefferey Steele, Van Zant , Columbia Records, 2005

{5} www.caregiver.org/making-end-life-decisions-what-are-your-important-papers

{6} "Phenomenon" 1996 Directed by Jon Turteltaub, written by Gerald Di Pego, and starring John Travolta.

{7} Saturday Night Live "Debbie Downer" played by Rachel Dratch, 2004 NBC Television

{8} "You've Got a Friend" written by Carole King, 1971 album Tapestry. Warner Bros. Records

More great sites for patients and caregivers:
www.cancer.org The American Cancer Society
www.abta.org American Brain Tumor Association
www.braintumornetwork.org Brain Tumor Network

~~~

As a companion to this book, and for your small groups at church, public and private groups, Charlie and Sherri have created a 7-part series titled "The Survivor Sessions". It is a Bible based program for the patients and caregivers, together and apart. For more details on how you can implement The Survivor Sessions in your area, email your location and contact information as well as any questions to: CharlieMarengo@gmail.com

Charlie and Sherri Marengo live in Petal, Mississippi, where they raised the 3rd and 4th generations of marching band kids. Now in his 14th year of 'remission', Charlie volunteers to counsel with anyone diagnosed with a brain tumor. They are members of Petal Harvey Baptist Church and spend lots of Saturdays traveling to the coast to soak up the sun.

In their semi-retirement, Charie ministers to people as the shuttle driver at the local hospital, while Sherri teaches acting to senior adults. They both love to share their testimony and sing and currently, are down to one chihuahua, Millie Blu- and that's enough!

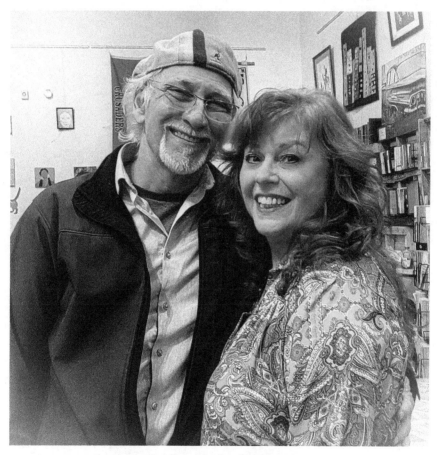

Charlie and Sherri Marengo